Childhood Encopresis and Enuresis

Causes and Therapy

Childhood Encopresis and Enuresis

Causes and Therapy

Charles E. Schaefer, Ph.D.

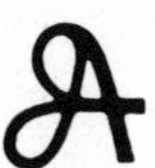

JASON ARONSON INC.
Northvale, New Jersey
London

1996 Softcover Edition

Library of Congress Cataloging in Publication Data

Schaefer, Charles E.
Childhood encopresis and enuresis.

Bibliography: p.
Includes index.
1. Encopresis in children. 2. Constipation in children. 3. Enuresis. 4. Toilet training.
I. Title.
RJ456.E48S3 618.9′23′42 79-9995
ISBN 1-56821-073-6

Manufactured in the United States of America. Jason Aronson Inc. offers books and cassettes. For information and catalog write to Jason Aronson Inc., 230 Livingston Street, Northvale, New Jersey 07647.

To my children, Karine and Eric,
who taught me a great deal about toilet training.

Preface

Childhood encopresis and enuresis have been a source of concern to many parents for over a millennium. Unfortunately, parents tend to know little about the causes or effective treatments for these disorders so they follow folklore rather than sound scientific advice.

In general, good advice does not include assuring the parents that their child will "grow out of" these disorders. It is true that, in time, most children do cease these problems on their own account. But this is often after years of living with a sense of failure, shame, embarrassing situations, intense parent-child conflicts, and often extreme and punitive forms of punishment. There are few things so deleterious to normal emotional development as the repeated and persistent failure, shame, and humiliation that many incontinent children feel. Also, it is a fact that some children *never* just outgrow these problems. The adverse effect on a child's psychosocial development of living with elimination problems for an extended period has been repeatedly noted. Children with persistent elimination disorders that are not treated tend to remain preoccupied with problems that other children have long since solved, so that these disorders interfere with learning, the development of friendships, and more mature personality development.

Mastery of bowel and bladder control is a major developmental milestone for children. This mastery represents a significant step towards the establishment of individuation. It signifies the ability to take care of oneself and attend school. Apart from lowering a child's self-esteem and causing social problems, elimination disorders are often reported to be the cause of child abuse incidents. A good example of the lack of parental tolerance for these disorders is the finding[1] regarding nonaccidental injury to children: next to crying, incontinence has emerged as the second most commonly stated reason for assaults.

Notwithstanding child abuse, persistent elimination problems in children produce parental guilt over not being effective parents, and worry that the child may be emotionally disturbed or never get over the problem.

Although many questions remain unanswered about childhood encopresis and enuresis, the extensive research conducted over the last 45 years has produced a growing awareness among professionals and the general public that most cases of persistent incontinence in children are primarily psychological in origin.

Until relatively recently, both enuresis and encopresis were conditions notoriously resistant to therapeutic intervention. Now, however, highly effective intervention techniques have been identified for these disorders and are becoming more widely used. But there is still a need for improved dissemination of knowledge about effective treatments, and for a greater number of qualified professionals to provide treatment for these disorders.

The purpose of this book is to provide the reader with a comprehensive overview of the causes, signs and effective treatments for childhood encopresis and enuresis. It is hoped that this book will stimulate greater interest, research and successful treatment of these disorders.

The book is divided into two major parts: the first section dealing with childhood encopresis and constipation, and the second section with enuresis. The data in this book are primarily based upon findings from journal articles in the world literature, together with the author's extensive experience in treating encopretic and enuretic children in a variety of settings. The bibliographies at the end of each section contain over 100 references to both original and review articles published in English and foreign languages, and are meant to be comprehensive rather than exhaustive. Glossaries of terms are also included to assist nonprofessionals in understanding the technical language contained in this volume.

[1]Kempe, C.H. and Helfer, R.E. *Helping the battered child and his family*. Oxford, England, Lippincott, 1972.

A basic premise of this book is that we need, at times, to curb our tendency to encompass the whole spectrum of children's psychosomatic disorders at one time, and content ourselves with smaller slices of knowledge so as to make more progress with specific disorders. According to Ruesch,[2] more in-depth studies of a single disorder can lead to greater understanding and treatment effectiveness. Psychosomatic disorders, in particular, tend to be quite complex, involving numerous systems such as somatic, cognitive, emotional and social.

This handbook is written primarily for professionals who work with children, including nurses, pediatricians, psychologists and social workers. It should also be of interest to parents and child care workers who wish to understand and help their encopretic and/or enuretic children. Moreover, teachers and students in courses on child therapy, child management or childhood psychopathology will find this book to be a valuable supplementary text.

[2]Ruesch, J. Psychosomatic medicine and the behavior sciences. *Psychosomatic Medicine,* 1961, 23, 277–286.

Charles E. Schaefer

Contents

Childhood Encopresis and Enuresis

Causes and Therapy

Part I
Childhood Encopresis

1

Introduction

Persistent fecal soiling can result in a virtual pariah status for the school-age child. The problem brings ridicule and shame to the child, evokes feelings of anger, disgust and guilt in the parents, embarrasses the family members, annoys educators and confounds therapists. Moreover, the problem often leads to child abuse by parents. The foul odor of feces is something adults and children alike find it extremely difficult to tolerate.

The usual response an ecopretic child elicits from otherwise imperturbable professionals is one of futility, prudishness, contempt and eagerness to pass the child and the problem along to someone else. An attitude of hopelessness has tended to prevail as the norm in dealing with this problem.[1]

Unfortunately, people are still embarrassed when discussing bowel movements. One of the most essential of all bodily functions, then, is still a taboo topic and is often made the subject of crude and vulgar "bathroom" humor. This attitude results in the fact that encopresis and constipation are often poorly treated, if treated at all. It is hoped that this book will contribute to a greater realization that encopresis and childhood constipation are serious problems that deserve and demand more widespread professional and public attention. A basic assumption of this book is that social ostracism, scapegoating, and physical abuse of an encopretic child are inversely related to the advancement of clinical knowledge and education of the public.

Childhood encopresis and constipation are disorders that have received relatively little professional and public interest until recently.

[1]Baird, M. *Bulletin of the Menninger Clinic,* 1974, 38, 144.

Indeed, encopresis and constipation were childhood disorders that parents and professionals were least likely to talk about and least likely to be effective in treating. In this regard, Anthony (1957) said,

> "Clinicians on the whole, perhaps out of disgust, prefer neither to treat them [encopretics] nor to write about them. The literature as compared with enuresis is surprisingly scanty . . . and superficial." (p.157)

Within the past 10 years, however, there has been a marked upsurge in research and clinical interest and activity in this area. As a result there are now a number of treatment strategies that have proven successful in eliminating these most distressing childhood disorders within a relatively short period of time. A treatment plan which combines behavioral methods (rewards and penalties) with pharmacological intervention has proven most effective. The goal of this section is to present a comprehensive survey of the latest findings concerning the origins, effect, and treatment of childhood encopresis and constipation.

DEFINITIONS AND DIAGNOSIS

Encopresis can be defined as repeated, involuntary defecation into clothing (or other unusual receptacle), occurring in children four years or older and of at least one month's duration. *Psychogenic* encopresis refers to the majority of cases of encopresis which are functional in nature, that is, they have no apparent organic or physiological causes in the usual sense, but are based on one or more of a number of factors including emotional disturbance, failure to develop a regular pattern for defecation, improper diet and so on. Psychogenic encopresis should be distinguished from neurogenic and anatomic megacolon. *Neurogenic Megacolon* or Hirschsprung's disease results from an absence of both ganglion cells and normal peristaltic waves in the bowel. Evacuation of colon is very difficult for these children and it is not unusual for them to have only one bowel movement a month. This condition must be corrected surgically. *Anatomic Megacolon* is a condition resulting from obstructing lesions or tumors in the bowel. A medical examination is needed to diagnose these cases.

In *Primary* encopresis bowel control was never attained, while in *Secondary* encopresis the child regressed to soiling after having established sphincter control for a period of time.

To assist the reader in making a differential diagnosis between psychogenic and neurogenic encopresis, Table 1 presents the important differentiating features between the two disorders. Table 1 is adapted from Garrard and Richmond (1952).

The first case of psychogenic or emotionally caused fecal soiling was reported by Fowler (1882). In this case a seven-year-old boy had ambitious parents who had pushed him prematurely into a rigorous educational schedule. The term encopresis was first used by Weissenberg (1926) to describe emotionally caused fecal soiling. Children with psychogenic encopresis usually soil their underwear

TABLE 1. Differential Diagnosis.

Psychogenic Megacolon	Neurogenic Megacolon
Admitting complaint:	Admitting complaint:
Fecal soiling	Constipation without fecal soiling
Age at onset:	Age at onset:
Second year or later	Birth or first weeks of life
History:	History:
Coercive bowel training	Lack of coercive bowel training (enemas only for true obstipation)
Toilet training successful at some time or always unsuccessful	Toilet training usually successful
Infrequent use of toilet after onset	Use of toilet for defecation
Defecation in standing or supine position	Defecation in sitting position
Inhibition of stool	Rarely abdominal pain
Colicky abdominal pain	Pellet-like or ribbon-like stools
Periodic voluminous stools	
Past History:	Past History:
No episodes of intestinal obstruction	Frequent episodes of intestinal obstruction
Physical examination:	Physical examination:
Feces-packed rectum	Empty rectum
Fluoroscopy (Neuhauser's technic):	Fluoroscopy (Neuhauser's technic):
Absence of spastic segment of rectum or rectosigmoid	Presence of spastic segment of rectum or rectosigmoid
Course:	Course:
Negligible mortality	High mortality if untreated

from once to several times each day – typically in the late afternoon – with a moderate amount of feces. When severe constipation is present, a small amount of greenish, mucoid, fetid material – produced by irritation of the rectal wall, is passed several times a day. Typically, the school-age child doesn't appear to be bothered by encopresis, although it generally infuriates his or her parents. This disorder occurs infrequently during school but commonly in play after school.

Constipation may be defined as a dysfunction in which the bowels are evacuated either at long intervals, with difficulty, or both. Hard, dry stools which are difficult to pass are common. Constipation may be due to several self-induced reasons such as low intake of food, low intake of fiber-containing foods, lack of exercise, and ignoring the urge to defecate; it may also result from environmental factors such as poor toilet facilities, travel or hospital admission.

INCIDENCE

An encopretic incidence of 1.5 percent is reported among seven to eight-year-old children of the Western world. Thus, a sizable number of children have had this little publicized disorder. Encopretic children are predominantly boys (ratio of 3.5 to 1) and generally, the first-born sons. This finding is in keeping with the usually higher frequency of problem behaviors and subtle neurological difficulties in boys. Paradoxically, constipation is more commonly reported in girls.

The incidence ratio of Hirschsprung's disease to psychogenic megacolon is quite small, that is, about 1:20.

Encopresis is largely a condition of prepubertal children, ages three to eleven, since it tends to resolve itself in adolescence. It declines spontaneously with age at a rate of 28 percent per year, virtually disappearing by age sixteen. Consequently, the long-term prognosis of encopresis is good, even without treatment, although it may last two or three years before it disappears. With treatment it often improves within a few weeks and disappears by two or three months. It is rare in adolescents and young adults except in severely retarded or psychotic persons.

In most cases, a physical examination of encopretic children reveals no anatomical or neurological difficulty, although dilation of the lower colon may be present as a result of retained feces. Thus, the majority of encopretic cases in childhood seem to be psychogenic in nature.

ETIOLOGY OF PSYCHOGENIC ENCOPRESIS

Among the causes of childhood encopresis that have been reported in the literature are the following:

1. Physiological Factors

Physiological problems are probably present when fecal retention and constipation are reported. Some children are reported to have constipation problems related to constitutional predisposition. When fecal matter is retained so as to stretch the bowel, excessive drying of the stool results and a hard impaction is present.

Constipation can result from a faulty diet (insufficient bulk or insufficient fluids), or from children who voluntarily inhibit defecation due to a previous history of painful lesions at the anus or because of social necessity due to late rising. A school-age child in a hurry to catch the school bus in the morning may avoid taking time for normal defecation. A child involved in outside play after school may also disregard the urge to defecate.

Failure to establish a regular, definte schedule for defecation may also be an important element. When this is combined with a relatively sedentary way of life, or a diet of soft, low-residue foods, it is easy to understand why a child may develop a "lazy" colon.

2. Social Interaction

Parental attitudes and toilet training habits are frequently mentioned in the genesis of encopresis. Parents with coercive or overly zealous toilet training strategies often trigger a tug-of-war with the child over this issue. Much hostility results on both sides, and the child unconsciously uses encopresis as a way of infuriating and tormenting his or her parents who cannot enforce obedience in this regard. Parents who are too concerned about cleanliness and regularity of bowel movements tend to over-use laxatives and enemas, both of which contribute to a lack of control in a child.

Bowel control usually comes after a child can walk—somewhere between one and two-and-a-half years of age.

When bowel training is initiated relatively late, the total time required to complete the training has been found to be less. Thus, when parents began bowel training before the child was five months old, nearly ten months (on the average) were required for success. However, when training was started later (20 months or older), only about five months were required.

When toilet training is initiated at too early an age, it often leads to constipation in later life. Most pediatricians agree that 15 months is the earliest age at which toilet training should be started.

Another type of faulty toilet training involves the parent who is lax to the point of indifference. In this case the child fails to develop regular toileting habits which can lead to a general lack of concern about being clean.

3. Situational Stress

Stress due to external events are frequently mentioned as contributing factors to encopresis. Sources of stress include birth of a sibling, loss of a parent due to death, divorce, or desertion, or starting school. Emotional causes are always expressed through the autonomic nervous system. In most cases the colon will be involved because it is well known to be one of the most nervous organs in the body (nervous tension often produces diarrhea or constipation). In regard to constipation, prolonged nervous tension can result in a chronic spastic condition in the colon (steady and prolonged contraction of the colon muscles) which not only inhibits the normal passing of stools but leads to drying out of the fecal mass.

4. Personality Correlates

Many authors refer to the following behavior traits of encopretic children:

shy and withdrawn
obedient and conforming
nonassertive and anxiety-prone
stoic, immature, and obstinate or stubborn
depressed

Many encopretic children appear to have temperaments described as "slow-to-warm-up," characterized by fear of new situations or novel experiences. Since shyness tends to be such a prominent feature they tend to be governed by fears which inhibit their range of options. A child like this may hold back defecation when forced to use strange toilet facilities.

Others find associated behavior such as immaturity, motor incoordination, enuresis and language difficulty.

Encopretic children often display a stoical attitude toward their condition, cloaking their anxiety with indifference. They tend to keep their feelings bottled up inside as they do their feces. Commonly described as passive, withdrawn, and obstinate, these children frequently express a total lack of awareness of, or concern about, their fecal soiling.

5. Genetic Factors

A greater history of childhood soiling by the parents and relatives of encopretic children has been reported. This suggests some genetic predisposition towards this particular disorder. About one-fourth of children with encopresis *have regular* problems with constipation which also suggests a constitutional or genetic predisposition.

In summary, psychogenic encopresis results from a complex interaction of many factors, such as genetic, physiological, psychological, interactional and cultural. It would seem then, that the most effective treatment approach is a holistic one that takes into account all of these etiological factors.

2

Bowel Physiology

An understanding of normal bowel anatomy and physiology is essential for effective treatment of encopresis. To recognize and help children with this disorder we must first understand the mechanism by which the body digests food and eliminates waste products.

DIGESTIVE SYSTEM

The gastrointestinal tract is phylogenetically the oldest system in the body, and hence it is the one most likely to be used to express an emotion which cannot be coped with through the regular channels. When a child's needs such as loving and being loved, being protected, are frustrated or not successfully carried out, this oldest system of the body may be used to express the problem. This has been called "organ language." Since it is not intended for service of this nature, especially for extended periods, such GI tract expression causes dysfunction and discomfort which results in physical problems in this area.

The GI tract is characterized by three different physiological functions: motility, vascularity, and secretion. From a normal baseline of activity, these three functions may vary in either an overactive or an underactive direction. Overactivity leads to hypermotility, vascular engorgement, and excessive secretion; underactivity leads to hypomotility, vascular pallor, and minimal secretion. In general, these three states are mediated through the rich innervation of the GI tract with both sympathetic and parasympathetic paths of the autonomous nervous system.

Experimental studies (Chapman and Loeb, 1955) have shown that the most significant factors in changing the states of motility, vascularity, and secretion seem to be emotional ones. These three functions may change rapidly, within minutes, depending on the emotional state of the child. Feelings of intense anxiety, unexpressed or unaware anger and resentment, and frustrated needs for affection may lead to hypermotility, hypervascularity and hypersecretion. On the other hand, feelings of depression, loneliness and isolation, and apathy may lead to hypomotility, hypovascularity, and hyposecretion. Hypoactivity of these three functions in the upper GI tract can lead to lack of appetite and severe weight loss, whereas hypoactivity of the lower GI tract can produce constipation.

A diagram of the gastrointestinal tract is presented in Figure 1. From the stomach the food mass, now thoroughly mixed with gastric juices and called chyme, enters the duodenum—the first part of the small intestine. It takes about 3½ to 5 hours for the liquid chyme to traverse the 23 feet of small intestine. Digestion is almost complete by the time the chyme leaves the small intestine and passes into the colon. By this time, the material which has not been digested in the small intestine is in a semiliquid state. Much of this liquid, together with some undigested nutrients, is absorbed by the large intestine. The remainder is formed into feces or waste material. The longer the feces remain in the large bowel, the drier they become because of the continual absorption of water. It takes about 12 to 18 hours for the material to traverse the 4 to 6 feet of large intestine.

The passage of food through the digestive tract is the result of a series of wavelike motions of the entire tract, termed peristaltic contractions. During each contraction the intestine above the food mass contracts and the portion of the intestine below the food mass relaxes, thus propelling the mass through the intestines towards the rectum.

When foods or liquids are swallowed a peristaltic "rush" begins in the upper intestinal tract and moves in a wave down to the rectum, forcing the bowel contents into the rectum. Distention of the rectum by the arrival of additional fecal material creates the urge-to-defecate sensation referred to as the "call to stool." When this urge is obeyed, contraction of the muscles of the pelvic floor causes another series of impulses which stop the movements of the colon and rectum,

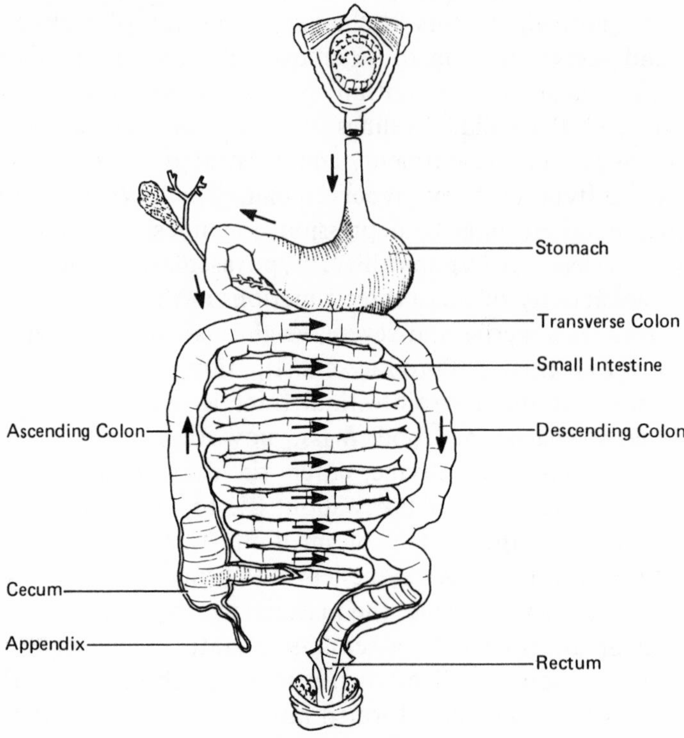

Figure 1. Diagram of Gastrointestinal Tract.

relax the sphincter muscle at the outlet of the rectum, and allow the stool to pass through. In most cases the strong peristaltic rush occurs daily and is strongest about 20 to 30 minutes after breakfast. This is not a hard and fast rule, however, and some people experience the peristaltic rush after each meal.

Peristalsis occurs in the colon, but not so frequently as it is observed in the small intestine, and mass movements occur at relatively infrequent intervals. These mass movements in the colon occur usually after a meal or intake of fluid. This increase in colonic motor activity is termed the gastrocolonic reflex. It has also been noted that prior to colonic activity, the terminal ileum becomes hyperactive following food or fluid intake, this activity being called the gastroileal reflex (Young, 1973). The mass movements of the colon empty the contents of the proximal colon into the more distal portions, and frequently such movements are followed by the desire to defecate.

On the average, three-quarters of food waste is excreted in 96 hours, but wide individual differences prevail here also. Most people have a bowel movement every day. Only about 1 percent of the normal population have an action less frequently than three times a week or more frequently than three times a day.

If for any reason defecation is prevented when the "call to stool" is present, the fecal mass is reposited into the sigmoid (lower end of colon) by means of reverse peristalsis. When this process is repeated many times the normally empty rectum tends to become accustomed to the presence of stool. If this occurs the stool will remain in the rectum without imparting a desire for defecation and *rectal constipation* is present. The term "constipation" is a relative one since it is entirely normal for some individuals to move their bowels only two or three times a week. Thus, absence of a daily movement does not in itself signal constipation. Constipation is not present if the stool is soft, moist on the outside surface, has a distinct shape, and if there is a feeling of emptiness of the rectum after defecation. If the stool is hard and dry, and there is a sense of incomplete evacuation, the child is constipated no matter how many times a day the bowel is moved.

TYPES OF CONSTIPATION

Three types of constipation not due to physical factors have been identified.

1. Rectal Constipation

This is the result of continued failure to obey the impulse to defecate. The child engrossed in play for example, may not respond to the "call to stool." Consequently, the rectum becomes "tolerant" of the increased pressure and amount of fecal matter it contains, and the urge to defecate passes. In the meantime, the colon is constantly absorbing water from its contents and the stool becomes hard, dry, and difficult to pass. Children, in particular, are reluctant to expel hard, large stools which are painful. Also, the water absorbing capacity of the rectum becomes impaired when it is impacted so that some watery stools may begin to leak out. In this condition there is a frequent release of watery stools but the child is really constipated.

2. Atonic Constipation

This is characterized by passage of hard, dry stools without accompanying abdominal pain. In this type of constipation the muscles of the colon have lost some of their ability to move the feces to the rectum. In large measure, atonic constipation seems to be caused by the long standing and excessive use of external cleansing agents (laxatives and enemas) which eventually tend to weaken the colon muscles.

3. Spastic Constipation

This is marked by constipation together with abdominal pain. The pain is caused by a spasm or involuntary contraction of the muscles of the colon. This condition is *by far* the most common form of constipation and is almost always due to emotional factors. Under periods of stress, people sometimes develop constipation characterized by the passage of small, hard stools, a lack of appetite, a lazy feeling, and mild abdominal pain.

Some people still believe that if feces are retained in the bowels for an extended period, poisons are absorbed into the body from them. This "autointoxication" theory has been proven to be a myth, together with the need for "daily regularity" which some laxative producers try to instill in the public. What may happen, since the rectum is very sensitive to pressure, is that a rectum disturbed due to a fecal mass may produce symptoms of headache, feelings of ill health, mental haziness, restlessness, irritability, or apathy.

ENEMAS

Since a constipated child with impacted feces has lost the normal urge to defecate and normal muscle tone in the colon, some external aid in relieving the fecal impaction should generally be given. When a child is constipated there is one procedure that not only helps empty the rectum but is both safe and effective—the enema. Unlike laxatives which take up to 12 hours to act, the enema acts immediately, and it does not affect the stomach or the upper intestinal tract.

1. Cleansing Enema

This is a solution of water, with certain additives, which is designed to empty the rectum (and sometimes the descending colon). The Fleet enemas available in most drugstores without a prescription are excellent cleansing enemas. The child size Fleet enema contains 2½ ounces of a fluid solution containing various salts, and is designed to penetrate the fecal mass quickly with fluid and increase the bulk volume of the rectum which in turn promotes the emptying of the feces in the rectum. Thus the enema imitates the normal stimulus for defecation by distending the rectum with the fluid. In general, 1 ounce of enema solution is used for every 20 pounds of a child's weight, with a maximum of 4½ ounces. Often a second enema is needed about an hour after the first. Usually you have to give more than one enema in the morning and at night to initially clean out a child with an impacted mass of feces in both the rectum and the bowel near the rectum. Never use plain water or soapsuds enemas. The Fleet enema contains both the liquid solution and the simple bulb syringe required for the administration.

Administration of Enemas

a. Have the child bend over in front of the toilet or lie on a bed, with knees drawn up, on top of a rubber sheet or bath towel.
b. Lubricate the bulb tip and the anus with vasoline jelly, insert the top gently for about one inch, and slowly squeeze the solution into the rectum. In a very short time the liquid will create a sense of distention which will lead to a desire to defecate. Promptly, withdraw the syringe and encourage a bowel movement after a few minutes. The water and whatever stool is in the rectum will be passed in the toilet.

Despite its simplicity, the enema is often performed improperly. Some cautions to follow are:

a. Don't introduce the fluid too rapidly. It can disturb the rectum and be quite painful. Rapid insertion will also stimulate the urge to defecate immediately so that the child cannot retain the fluid long enough for it to penetrate the feces.

b. Don't use soapy water which can irritate the rectal lining.
c. Avoid too rapid a flow of liquid, and stop the flow as soon as the pressure produces pain or marked discomfort. If discomfort is reported, have the child rest for a time and do not resume the flow until the discomfort disappears. Have the child retain whatever quantity of the enema that can be comfortably held. Repeat the procedure throughout the day until the rectal flow is clear.
d. Be sure to administer the enema in a calm manner without any display of negative emotions (such as disgust, impatience, anxiety, worry, uncertainty, hostility, and so on). Be supportive, friendly, understanding, and encouraging to the child.
e. Remember that the rectum is very sensitive to pressure. When disturbed as a result of enemas and fecal matter it may produce the following symptoms in certain children: headaches, feeling of being sick, pain, mental haziness, dizziness, nausea. Be on the lookout for any signs of these disorders.
f. Before giving an enema be sure to prepare the child for the experience by describing in simple terms the purpose, procedure, and the sensations (e.g. mild unpleasantness) or feelings (e.g. embarrassment) that it is likely to produce. Enlist the child's cooperation and tell about each step as you go along. Ask the child to take deep breaths to relax the anus and rectum and then insert the lubricated rectal tube slowly and gently. Be sure the child is in the supine or prone position so that the fluid can reach the colon. Have the child maintain the position after inserting the solution until the urge to defecate is strong (usually within 1 to 5 minutes).
g. Prior to an enema have the child void if possible since an empty bladder reduces pressure within the abdominal cavity.
h. Be sure to note the results of one enema—the color, amount, and consistency of the stool.
i. Wash your hands before and after the procedure.

2. Lubricating Enemas

These involve the insertion of mineral or olive oil into the rectum by a simple bulb syringe to soften the feces and lubricate the anal passage. Often the oil is introduced at night into the rectum and expelled the following morning either naturally or with the help of a cleansing enema.

Glycerine suppositories are easier to administer than a lubricating enema and are intended to serve the same purpose, namely to soften, lubricate, and stimulate evacuation. Unfortunately, glycerine suppositories have resulted in only limited success in evacuating hard feces in children and adults.

One method of bowel evacuation employs the quick-acting suppository bisacodyl (Dulcolax) which is inserted in the rectum once daily for three days according to a predetermined schedule (Halpern and Kissel, 1976). Since evacuation occurs within half an hour after insertion, the child can be prepared to anticipate successful movement into the toilet without the more intrusive effect of an enema. Also, older children are able to insert this suppository themselves. An occasional side effect on the first try is abdominal cramping which may require reassurance as to its transient nature.

After three days use the child is encouraged to have bowel movements without the use of the suppository. Should the child develop retention again for a three-day period, the Dulcolax suppository is again employed for three days to prevent the recurrence of constipation. In this way the child comes to expect that bowel elimination can be brought under his or her control and regular bowel habits are reestablished.

LAXATIVES

Although laxatives can and do help the colon discharge retained feces and thus temporarily relieve constipation, they do so at the expense of irritating the colon, reducing the ability of the colon to do its own work, and increasing the likelihood the user will become dependent on the laxative habit.

The types of laxatives include:

1. Bulk Products

These are basically indigestible substances. They work by irritating the lining of the bowels high up, and thereby force waste out.

2. Mineral Oils and Emulsions

These are designed to produce cylindrical, easily passed stools. However, they can cause nausea, anal leakage, loss of fat-soluble vitamins, and prevent absorption of food nutrients by coating the intestines.

3. Chemical Irritants

These include senna and cascara and they can be extremely dangerous if tight, tense colonic muscles are present. By overstimulating tense muscles they can worsen spastic constipation.

4. Saline Products

Milk of magnesia, epsom salts, and sodium phosphate act by preventing the absorption of water in the stomach so that more fluids reach the colon and rectum. Frequent use of these products, however, can seriously disturb the normal digestive process by neutralizing the digestive acids of the stomach.

The use of laxatives to treat childhood encopresis and constipation is not recommended because of their possible adverse effect on the digestive system. The first principle in bowel management which appears from all the recent advances in knowledge, is the need to leave the complex mechanisms of the gastrointestinal tract as undisturbed as possible. The best laxatives are the natural ones contained in a proper diet of fruits, vegetables, and plenty of water.

DIET

Improper diets can contribute to the development and maintenance of constipation and encopresis in children. Certain foods have a binding effect on the gastrointestinal system and should be restricted when a child is constipated, while others have a natural laxative effect on the GI tract. Large amounts of the following foods can have a binding effect: cheese, milk, butter, fatty meats, egg yolk, and "junk" food such as chocolate bars, cookies, coke.

Foods with high bulk or fiber content tend to retain water longer and produce softer stools of good size, weight, and consistency.

They result in a more rapid transit rate through the GI tract (by increased peristalsis) and a much stronger "call to stool." Examples of fiber containing food products are fruits (apples, bananas, peaches, prunes, figs, raisins, berries, and melons); vegetables (lettuce, spinach, cabbage, carrots, cauliflower, asparagus, tomatoes, sweet corn, and sweet potatoes); and grain (whole wheat cereals, graham crackers, brown and whole grain breads).

It is also important for free elimination to drink plenty of fluids (four to six glasses of water a day). By drinking plenty of water you help to reduce dry stools. Milk, because of its binding effect is best kept to one pint a day when one is constipated. Many doctors recommend that the child drink a glass of hot water laced with lemon juice upon arising, since this serves to stimulate the gastrocolonic reflex.

In general one should strive for a dietary happy medium. Some bulk foods are good but a continuous eating of figs, shredded wheat and bran can cause inflammation of the bowel and spastic constipation. When a nervous or spastic colon is present, roughage should be reduced and a bland diet introduced to relieve the already overactive sigmoid colon of the extra stimulation of roughage. To prevent constipation the diet should be high in proteins, low in carbohydrates, and low in fats.

Some other guidelines in regard to a child's diet are as follows:

Do have the child eat at regular times and about the same amount of food every day at each meal. If more food than usual is consumed at a meal, or if mealtime is haphazard, the natural rhythm of the body for digesting and evacuating food is disturbed. So establish a daily schedule for meals and encourage the child to eat about the same amount at each meal.

Do consult your physician about the proper diet for a constipated child.

Do encourage a child to chew the food well since poorly masticated food puts a strain on the GI system and can lead to constipation.

EXERCISE

Physical activity has been found to encourage the onward propulsion of bowel waste. So regular exercise will help promote bowel movements in children. The sedentary or inactive child, on the other hand, will be more prone to constipation difficulties.

DRUGS

Musicco (1977) successfully treated an eight-year-old boy with encopresis (total incontinence of liquid or soft excreta, partial control of solid excreta) by administering a drug containing adenosine and organic phosphoric acid initially, and then the drug UTP (uridine-5-triphosphate). The latter seemed to act on the musculature of the lower bowel, producing an increase in contractions and muscle activity. Rectal exam prior to treatment had revealed a slight hypotonia of the anal sphincter muscle.

Some authors report medication effective for nonretentive encopresis (Halpern, 1977). Fowler (1882) advocated antispasmodics such as belladonna to control fecal soiling. More recently, imipramine (Tofranil) has been used by Abrahams (1963) and Gavanski (1971) but the rationale and site of action has not been clear.

3

Toilet Training Practices and Childhood Encopresis-Constipation

An analysis of childrearing advice to American parents since the turn of the century reveals dramatic shifts in approach. In the early 1900s a permissive infant care approach prevailed, while the twenties and thirties witnessed a radical shift to strict toilet training (high control, close monitoring, rigid scheduling), then a return to a more indulgent "child-oriented" approach in the forties and fifties occurred and, finally, the current pluralistic diversity of childrearing advice emerged. Each change has mirrored the mood and pressure of historical events and has been stimulated by the results of the latest scientific investigation. The two key aspects of toilet training involve how early it should begin, and how severe or pressured it should be.

The more severe the training procedure and the earlier it is initiated, the more upset the child is likely to be by the training, with severity being the important aspect. A large number of children with bowel and bladder dysfunction have been found to have experienced very early and/or very severe training regimes. Bemporad *et al.* (1971), for example, found that 11 of 14 encopretic children were trained before they were 18 months old. Many studies reveal even earlier training which tends to be rather severe or harsh.

HOW EARLY?

Some years ago 11 months was the average age for beginning bowel training in America. In the twenties and thirties it was even earlier.

According to Huschka (1942), a 1935 U.S. Children's Bureau publication on infant care stated:

> Training of the bowels may be begun as early as the end of the first month. It should always be begun by the third month and may be completed by the eighth month.

The writer went on to urge "absolute regularity" in providing this training, including "not varying the time by five minutes." Detailed instructions for "using the soap stick as an aid in conditioning the rectum" were also presented. Blatz and Bott (1929) advocated placing children on the pot during the third month at a regular time each day. A soap-stick or glycerine suppository was used to induce defecation. Typically it takes about seven months to complete training although some babies develop control within a few weeks, while others require a year-and-a-half or more.

Over the last four decades a gradual postponing of the initiation of bowel training has occurred (Caldwell, 1964). In the 1940s there was research suggesting that the cortical centers governing elimination do not begin to function before six months of age, making voluntary control before that time difficult if not impossible. Thus, Huschka (1942) recommended that parents should wait until eight months before beginning training.

Subsequently, Fraiberg (1959) stated that in order for a child to cooperate in his toilet training, he or she must be able to control the sphincter muscles, have the ability to postpone the urge to defecate, and be able to give a signal to be taken to the bathroom or get there on his/her own initiative. In normal child development, Fraiberg concluded that these conditions may not be present until 15 to 18 months or later. Most pediatricians today suggest four criteria for determining if a child is ready for toilet training:

1. Can the child sit firmly and securely on the seat?
2. Can the child retain the stool until placed on the seat?
3. Can the child communicate the need to defecate?
4. Does the child have an understanding of the social implications of defecation?

The current thinking is that at 18 months most children will physiologically and psychologically meet the above criteria. Thus, Brazelton

(1962) advises that after the age of 18 months, parents should gradually introduce their infant to the pot. Notice the time of day the child usually empties his/her bowels and place the child on the toilet at these times for five or ten minutes. Immediately praise any evacuations or attempts. Do not force the child to remain on the potty against his/her will. He urges an unpressured approach so as to facilitate the infant's autonomous control of elimination. Sphincter control at age two or three is considered a developmental task by most child development experts today. Ilg and Ames (1955) maintain that really consistent success in controlling the bowels should be expected by age two.

The sequence in the development of sphincter control is typically, but not always, as follows: the child first acquires control of the bowels while asleep, and then control of the bowels during waking hours. Control of the bladder while awake soon follows, and then, after a rather variable interval, control of the bladder while asleep. Children delayed in acquiring bowel control also tend to be delayed in acquiring bladder control. According to Stein and Susser (1967), control of the bowels by 18 to 24 months is typical in America. Control of the bladder during the day is acquired by most children by age four, control at night by age four-and-a-half years. Girls tend to be ahead of boys in both bowel and bladder control. According to the normal developmental sequence, then, a child signals readiness for daytime bowel training when there is regularity in bowel movements, and when control of the bowel while asleep is achieved.

The total time required to complete bowel training has been found to be less (as in the case of weaning) when it is initiated relatively late. When parents began bowel training before the child was five months old, nearly 10 months (on average) were required for success. But when training was begun later (at 20 months or older), only about five months were required (Sears, *et al.*, 1957). In this study, the middle-class children whose toilet training was begun between five and 14 months or after 19 months, manifested fewest emotional problems during training.

There are wide cultural variations in the time of beginning toilet training. Lower-class American parents tend to begin this training early, as do Europeans. In one cross-cultural study, the median age of starting regular toilet training in London was 4.6 months, in Paris 7.8 months, and in Stockholm 12.4 (Hindley *et al.*, 1965). Early toilet training in China is now reported to be the custom (Cohen, 1977), with most children achieving control of both feces and urine by 18 months. Gentleness and care rather than harshness seems to be the custom in training children now in the People's Republic of China.

Anthropologists have shown that a society's specific infant training practices are adaptive to survival and cultural values. Some primitive tribes are notoriously carefree about the whole business, while others start very early. deVries and deVries (1977) report on the East African Digo tribe which believes that infants can learn soon after birth, and begin motor and toilet training in the first weeks of life. With a nurturant conditioning approach by the mother, night and day dryness is achieved by most Digo children by five or six months. The success of early Digo training suggests that sociocultural factors are more important determinants of toilet training readiness than maturation of the nervous system. It would seem, then, that it is not how early one begins toilet training that is crucial (although later training tends to result in quicker and more efficient training), but how harsh or severe are the parents' attitudes and practices in this area.

HOW SEVERE?

Toilet training can become a major source of friction between parent and child, and a "battle of the bowel" can result. In such a battle the child learns to associate anxiety and/or disgust with toilet functions, which can result in efforts to avoid defecation and consequently, constipation and encopresis. On the other hand, parental neglect of toilet training can result in a general lack of concern by the child about being clean. Anthony (1957) associates this overly permissive approach, which leaves the learning of control almost entirely up to the child, with the continuous or primary type of encopresis (children who never had been trained), while he relates high anxiety and fear of being punished for "accidents" with secondary or discontinuous encopresis.

There is general agreement that a middle ground between the extremes of a harsh, punitive, rigid parental approach (that makes frequent use of shame, blaming, threats, punishment) and a lax, indifferent, laissez-faire approach (that gives little or no guidance to a child) is the best approach to toilet training. In other words, be temperate or moderate in your training. Also, toilet training is most likely to proceed both smoothly and quickly if the parents encourage the gradual acquisition of control.

TOILET-TRAINING GUIDELINES

A questionnaire survey (Benjamin *et al.*, 1971) of parents who had successfully toilet trained their children revealed that efficient toilet training was related to the following procedures: (1) the presence of a discriminative stimulus, such as switching from diapers at night to training pants or pajamas; (2) having a motivated, responsible child—for example, one parent said, "It was really the child's idea that it was time to begin night training"; (3) maximizing conditions to elicit the desired response—"I had him urinate immediately after he woke up in the morning"; and (4) rewarding success with positive reinforcers—"I said in a pleased manner, You can keep dry pants all by yourself." In addition, this study found that negative parental reinforcers, such as shaming, spanking, rejecting, and name calling, impeded night training.

It has been the author's experience that the following ten, simple elements will lead to effective toilet training for most children:

1. Attitude

The attitude of the parents during toilet training should be that of a teacher instructing a child in a new skill. Be calm, patient, gentle and encouraging. Failure to go on the pot should be accepted in a matter-of-fact manner and the child returned to his or her normal activity. Give no overt sign of disapproval for accidents or failure to defecate on the pot. Impart to the child the simple understanding that grown-ups use the toilet for elimination. Avoid irritation, scolding, or punishment. Be firm rather than forcing. Thus, do not force the child to remain on the seat for more than five to ten minutes or make the child feel guilty for noncompliance. Remember that the ability to retain the stool is learned earlier than the ability to release it at the right time. If a child has an accident a few minutes after potty training he or she is not being "hateful." Since no one learns a new skill all at once, expect mistakes and training lapses.

Remember the basic rule in toilet training: never make an issue of it. After all, you are dealing with an infant. *Patience* and a *matter-of-fact* attitude are the keys to your child's learning bowel and bladder control in an effective way.

Try to examine your own attitudes about bowel habits and understand how they may affect the child. Do you become emotionally upset about toilet training because you are overly concerned about regularity, cleanliness or obedience? Do you tend to be perfectionistic or competitive so that you drive your children towards more mature behavior at a faster pace than other parents?

2. Relationship

According to Anthony (1957), the key to effective toilet training is the parent-child relationship. In a warm, nurturing relationship, the child will do as the parent asks, not because the parent demands, threatens, or bribes, but because the child wants to please. In a similar vein, Woodmansey (1968) stated that a normal child in an ordinary home is eager to conform to the cultural patterns of the family as soon as he/she is able to do so, and will adopt the toilet habits when sphincter control is physically mature enough, and his/her life is not impaired by interpersonal friction or inner conflicts. An excellent way to build and maintain a relationship is to spend time alone with each child every day while engaged in mutually enjoyable activities.

If you encounter any training "problems" that upset you, or keep you from being on good terms with your child, set all training aside until you feel more relaxed about the whole thing. In the meantime, enjoy all the other things the child is learning, and let the child enjoy being a baby.

3. Equipment

Use a potty chair which offers good support (on the floor) for his/her feet and which is sturdy and comfortable so the child feels safe and secure. A toilet chair with arms, which sits on the floor over a potty, is likely to make the child feel more comfortable than the kind which rests on the adult seat. The floor provides the necessary "push" and foot support for good bowel action, and the child won't be frightened by the flushing of the toilet.

4. Routines

To promote regularity, establish consistent routines for a child's toileting. Toilet the child at a regular time each day. Since the peristaltic rush from mouth to rectum following intake of food is greatest after breakfast, try making a regular habit of a trip to the bathroom right after breakfast. Don't become so rigid about a child's toileting schedule that you can never vary it. Only place the child on the potty once, or at most, twice a day. Help your child become regular in all habits. This includes not only elimination and eating habits but exercise and sleeping habits.

In addition to fixed routines, be responsive to your child by watching for signs that the child needs to defecate (grunts, straining, crying, red in the face), and take the child to the bathroom immediately.

5. Discriminative Stimulus

After ascertaining that a child is ready to begin toilet training, inform the child that you believe he/she is now ready to take care of his/her own bowel movements and underclothes. In regard to bladder training, after the child shows his/her readiness by being regularly dry for two hours at a time, take him/her out of diapers and use training pants. The new pants will act as a stimulus to the child that different, more grown-up behavior is now expected.

6. Cueing or Prompting

By taking the child to the bathroom and placing him/her on the pot, you give the child visual cues that defecation is expected. You should also give a verbal cue by repeating the simple word you have chosen to call the act of defecation. At first you may have to signal the child to defecate by imitating the grunting, grimacing signs the child usually gives when defecating. In one way or another let the child know what is expected on the potty.

Don't wait until the child tells you he/she wants to defecate. Give gentle reminders to use the toilet during the early stages of toilet training. If this is done often, the connections between the pattern of intentional cues (bowel and bladder tensions) and the external cues (the bathroom), and the responses of excretion become strengthened.

7. Rewards

Success on the potty should be immediately praised. A simple edible treat like a cookie or candy might also be given in the beginning to motivate the child to try for self-control. Remember that positive reinforcement rather than punishment works best in toilet training. Don't overpraise. Simply smile and say "good."

8. Imitation

Try capitalizing on the child's natural tendency to imitate, by taking the child with you to the toilet and demonstrating the expected behavior, instructing the child to imitate you. In one African tribe some mothers, instead of teaching, simply tell the child to imitate what the older children do (LeVine and LeVine, 1963).

9. Individual Differences

Since some children mature later than others, parents need to have patience and accept the child's natural developmental patterns. If the initial few weeks of toilet training efforts are not successful or if the child strongly resists, the parents should wait until the child is four to six weeks older before trying again. Rather than initiate a power struggle over elimination, parents should leave the toilet training pretty much up to the child who will learn with very little trouble as soon as he or she is ready.

10. Rebellion

Occasionally a child may deliberately soil or resist training as a way of asserting independence. Try being less firm in your efforts for a few days. This usually solves the situation.

TOILET TRAINING INTERVENTION FOR ENCOPRESIS-CONSTIPATION

In treating childhood encopresis or constipation several therapists have used, as their main technique, the instruction of parents as to more effective toilet training practices. Following a moderate training philosophy, Mercer (1961) advocates the following toilet training procedure for children with psychogenic constipation. First, advantage should be taken of the normal gastrocolonic reflex. After breakfast each morning the child should be instructed to go to the bathroom and sit on the toilet. Clocklike regularity of this habit is encouraged. Often, the entire family will have to get up a little earlier than usual so that the child will have sufficient time to relax in the bathroom after breakfast and not neglect this habit in the rush to get to school. No particular coercion should be used in attempting to establish the daily habit. He/she is not forced to remain in the bathroom after breakfast for any specific time other than the few minutes needed to attempt to defecate. If the child has the urge to go at any other time during the day he is allowed to go. The occasion for having a bowel movement should no longer become the focus of the day's activities, the cause for celebration, of calling grandmother on the phone, but assumes the appropriate role of being taken for granted without special notice. When parents have a matter-of-fact attitude about it, the child is less likely to use this event as an attention-gaining mechanism. In the event the constipated child goes three or four days without a movement, Mercer suggests that he be given an enema at the customary time after breakfast.

Believing in a more intense and structured toileting procedure, Butler (1977) treated three cases of encopresis by using principles of overcorrection training (Azrin and Foxx, 1971) and positive practice (Azrin and Foxx, 1974). As compared to other techniques for eliminating soiling, the overcorrection and positive practice techniques are educational in nature and help the child practice the correct responses.

The positive practice technique herein reported (the extensive practice of competing, appropriate behavior whenever a child misbehaves) meant that whenever the children soiled they were required by their parents to practice rapidly going to the bathroom for a specified number of trials–in this study 10 times. The overcorrection technique which involved training for cleanliness required the child to change clothes whenever he soiled, to bathe, and then wash his soiled clothes. Frequent inspections for dry pants throughout the day were also conducted by the parents, and edible treats and/or verbal praise were given at these times when the child's pants were not soiled. Each day the parents gave a telephone report to the therapist regarding the number of accidents by the child and any difficulties encountered with the program. Detailed written instructions regarding the program had been given the parents prior to the intervention.

It should be noted that the cleanliness training described above is less aversive than the full cleanliness training (Foxx and Azrin, 1973b) procedure which involves forced cleaning of clothes by the child for 20 minutes and forced cleaning of the body in cold water for 20 minutes.

Butler (1977) reports a case study of a 28-month-old boy who had been bladder trained at 20 months but who continued soiling at home. A recent physical exam by a pediatrician was within normal limits. For the first week the parents were asked to record the time and location of each bowel movement. Thereafter, each bowel accident was followed by a verbal reprimand, training for cleanliness, and positive practice. The cleanliness training meant the child was required to clean his soiled undergarment for three minutes in a specially provided receptacle. After washing he had to squeeze it out and hang it up to dry. He was then to clean himself around the genital area and buttocks for three minutes. If the child failed to complete any of these tasks his parents placed their hands on the hands of the child to assist him in completing the instructions. After cleaning he was required to put on a clean pair of underpants and then positive practice was begun. Positive practice called for 10 rapidly conducted trips to the toilet, with two from the original place of the accident and the rest from different locations throughout the house or yard. The parents manually guided any action in opposition to the positive practice. They also ignored any whining or crying by the child and stated several times before each positive practice trial that he had to practice going quickly to the toilet because he had dirtied his pants. Inspections for dry pants were made several times per day before major activities such as meals and bedtime. If the child's pants were not soiled, verbal praise or edible treats were dispensed by the parents. After the boy had five accident-free days, positive practice was stopped, and any future accidents resulted only in a verbal warning and cleanliness training. The inspections for dry pants were performed daily seven times per day during the treatment and were slowly phased out during the follow-up period. After eight days on the program the boy achieved five accident-free days and had no further soiling during a six-month follow-up period. From the first day of the program he had appropriate self-initiated bowel eliminations.

Similar success was reported by Butler with two other encopretic children, ages three and five. Since these older children would often hide or sneak off to have their "accidents," the parents were instructed to handle these attempts by directly prompting the child to go to the toilet using manual guidance and to have the child remain there for five minutes. Also, with the five-year-old it was necessary to give a Fleet enema if he went for several days without an evacuation. On the basis of these cases and his clinical experience, Butler concludes that overcorrection techniques seem most appropriate for encopretic children who are seven years or younger. He recommends a point system for older children.

4

Treatment Approaches for Encopresis

The major treatment approaches for childhood encopresis are presented in this chapter. Among the schools of thought described are the behaviorial, psychoanalytic, family therapy, and comprehensive approaches.

BEHAVIORAL APPROACH

Social learning theorists and behavior therapists in particular have been applying learning techniques to encopresis by directly treating the "symptom" without regard to any possible underlying disturbance. The basic premise is that this deviant behavior is learned and not a symptom of some underlying conflict or disease process. Thus, correction of the problem should follow the same "laws" of learning that resulted in the acquisition of the soiling behavior.

The literature has to date shown that the application of operant techniques (rewards and/or penalties) has been quite successful in helping children gain voluntary control over their defecatory responses. Most often, systematic retraining or conditioning techniques involve the use of both rewards and penalties.

Rewards and Penalties

The use of rewards and penalties (carrot and stick approach) involves the application of external rewards for appropriate defecation and punishment for inappropriate defecation or soiling. This procedure makes it crystal clear to the child what the consequences will be for desired and undesired acts.

Houle (1974) combined positive reinforcement (rewards) for nonsoiling periods and aversive conditioning (punishments) for soiling incidents by a 12-year-old boy in residential treatment. He soiled at least once a day on average and many times twice a day. The plan was explained in detail to the child and his help and commitment to the program were solicited.

First, the child was given a monthly chart on which the days of the week were divided into two blocks, each block representing a half day. For each half day he went without soiling, he was given a gold star which he pasted on the respective half day block. Each time he was awarded a star he was also praised by the houseparent. For every two consecutive stars (a full day) he was given a special treat—generally a candy bar. While he ate the bar an adult would praise him and avoid any negative comments. Six consecutive stars enabled him to participate in a special activity such as bowling. For every ten consecutive stars the boy was allowed to go on an off-campus activity such as a fishing trip. The special treats and activities were changed every week so the child would not lose interest in the program.

The aversive task required the boy, as soon as he soiled himself, to take a shower, put on clean clothes and rinse the soiled clothes out in a tub. The rinsing task was inspected by a houseparent and the boy was informed that it was "okay" or "do it again." No scolding, special attention, or praise was given to the boy during this clean-up time. Indeed little or no verbal interaction by an adult (which can be reinforcing) was accorded the boy during this aversive period.

After six weeks the boy's soiling behavior ceased so he was required to have four consecutive stars before he earned a treat. After the 11th week of the program he was given a star only for a complete day of nonsoiling. At the beginning of the 20th week the rewards and penalties were eliminated except that he was given occasional verbal praise for periods of nonsoiling. From the 13th to the 23rd weeks no soiling was evident and he had only three soiling incidents during the four months after this period.

Ayllon, Simon and Wildman (1975) helped a separated mother eliminate soiling in her seven-year-old boy. During the preceding year the child had never gone an entire week without soiling himself at least two or three times a week. When he currently soiled himself in school he would come home, take a bath, rinse out his clothing, change clothes and then continue with his daily activities. The mother's only attempt to deal with the problem was to repeatedly urge the boy to remember to use the toilet. At the school's urging, the mother and the boy sought psychological help for the encopresis. The mother was instructed to post a chart and give the boy a star on the chart just before bedtime for each day he had not soiled himself. Seven consecutive stars would earn the boy an outing to the place of his choice, such as a trip to a hamburger place with his cotherapists. After four weeks the boy was no longer soiling himself, so therapy contacts were not needed and the mother administered the chart system and the outings herself, on a very informal basis. Three months later the child continued to show no sign of encopresis, but the mother still praised him for not soiling and gave him a special trip about every other week. The use of the chart and stars had been dropped by this time.

In another case, parents of a five-and-a-half-year-old retarded, hyperactive, "autistic" boy rapidly eliminated his soiling (he had never been toilet trained) by restraining the child in a chair facing a bare corner of his room for 30 to 45 minutes after every misplaced bowel movement (Barrett, 1969). He was also given his favorite chocolate cookies and praised lavishly right after—and only after—every bowel movement on the toilet. The necessity of being 100 percent consistent in administering these consequences, while avoiding spanking and screaming over soiling episodes, was stressed. This procedure rapidly eliminated the encopresis. When the boy later tried to withhold feces for several days the use of suppositories quickly ended this behavior.

The use of "full cleanliness training" in combination with positive reinforcement effectively stopped the encopresis of a retarded male after 16 weeks of treatment (Doleys and Arnold, 1975). Full cleanliness training, contingent on inappropriate soiling, requires the child to clean himself and his clothing. This procedure involved three steps: (1) parents expressed displeasure about the soiling; (2) the child was required to scrub his soiled underwear for at least 15 minutes; and (3) he was then required to bathe and clean himself. The child was not released from the cleaning task if he was crying or being disruptive when the required time elapsed. Such overcorrection, it is felt, teaches the child to assume responsibility for correcting inappropriate behavior, and serves as an adversive consequence that motivates the child to perform the appropriate behavior. In the present case the parents also assisted the six-year-old boy by checking his pants every 15 to 20 minutes and reinforcing him for clean pants, and by having the boy sit on the toilet each hour for about ten minutes and reinforcing him in any attempt to defecate. A chart was kept on the wall of the bathroom and the boy colored in one of ten squares following each bowel movement. Ten completed squares earned him a toy (later 20 squares were needed).

A 12-year-old girl with a history of chronic encopresis was treated by being given periods of isolation (30 minutes in her room) as a punishment for fecal soiling, and later, in addition, by relieving her of dishwashing chores when she did not soil (Edelman, 1971). The child and her mother were given forms at the beginning of therapy to record the time and place of each soiling episode, what the child was doing when the soiling occurred, and what the consequences were for soiling. The mother was instructed to check the child's undergarments at the end of the day to verify the frequency of soiling. The program produced virtual complete suppression of soiling. Bedwetting diminished more or less concomitantly with soiling although it was not specifically treated.

Jerry, a six-year-old first grader had been soiling for the past four months. His parents were advised to initiate the following program since spankings and medical help had proved ineffective (Plachetta, 1976). First they were to avoid displaying any overt disapproval of the soiling and to simply require the child to wash the soiled garments–not as "punishment" but as a means of accepting responsibility for his actions. Jerry and his parents also made a verbal contract whereby four times per day (morning, noon, after school, before bed) he was to go to the toilet and *attempt* to eliminate. Each 10 minute "attempt" was rewarded with a penny, while each "success" received a nickel. An emphasis was placed on "trusting" Jerry to report accurately. The first week on this procedure the boy had only two "accidents" both the result of forgetting to defecate at noon while in school. To prompt himself in school Jerry pasted a picture of a commode in his lunchbox.

The second week the boy soiled eight times, probably because his parents were paying less attention to his successes now. The following changes were then implemented: (1) his parents praised him every time they gave money for success; and (2) a self-charting system was instituted whereby Jerry was given colored paper and crayons to make his own chart. For every day free of soiling he was allowed to cut out and paste a star on the chart so as to display his accomplishments. Jerry rarely soiled after this procedure was initiated, and was totally free of soiling within six weeks. He now stated that "I don't have to be paid for going to the toilet," and the charting and reward system was gradually eliminated. Also noteworthy is the fact that while this program was in effect the boy's parents were counseled as to effective child rearing practices, particularly in ways to reduce tension and pressure on children.

Rewards

Sometimes rewards alone without any penalties are sufficient to control encopresis. Perdini and Perdini (1971) used a reward to help an 11-year-old boy who frequently defecated in class. His mother reported that he had never been toilet trained. Since the boy enjoyed reading, it was decided to reinforce soiling-free periods in the classroom with coupons he could use for book purchases. The boy could earn eight coupons a day; he needed 40 coupons to obtain his first book, 55 for the second book, and so on. The soiling was immediately eliminated by this reward procedure, and follow-up several months after the elimination of book coupons revealed only one accident.

Ashkenazi (1975) found that encopretic children fell in two types. The first type of child showed a phobic reaction to the toilet or potty by crying, clinging to the mother, and refusing to approach the toilet. These children had all experienced painful bowel movements as a result of constipation or diarrhea episodes earlier in life. This phobic reaction was deconditioned by having the child gradually approach the toilet while the mother reduced anxiety and reinforced closer approaches with rewards of candies, raisins, chocolate or a favored toy, until the child could sit comfortably on the toilet for three minutes. The mothers "played this game" with the child several times a day until the objective was achieved (no more than five days was needed in any case).

A second group of encopretic children was willing to sit on the toilet but they claimed that they "did not know" when fecal elimination was about to take place. With this group Ashkenazi had the mother give the child a glycerine suppository after a meal (to increase rectal distention as a cue for elimination in the toilet). The child was then sent to the toilet after 15 to 20 minutes and if evacuation took place, praised and given a small prize. If no soiling occurred that day, the child was again rewarded with praise and a prize before bedtime. The mothers were instructed to gradually fade out the use of prizes, and then to praise only occasionally for appropriate elimination. This procedure was found to be very successful for this type of child.

Concrete rewards made contingent upon appropriate toilet elimination were also employed by Neale (1963). He reports four cases of psychogenic encopresis in children ages seven to ten. Because the soiling was of long standing and resistant to other forms of treatment, the children were all inpatients at a psychiatric hospital. After each main meal and at bedtime, the children were taken to the toilet by a warm friendly nurse. The procedure was explained to the children and they were given comic books to read on the toilet if they wished. After successful passing of feces, the child was rewarded by adult approval and the knowledge of progress toward greater self-control. In addition, the children were given a reward of sweets, peanuts, pennies, or stars in a book. Two of the children were orally given a dried mucilage of tropical seeds that gave additional bulk for the colon to work on and made the stools soft and easy to pass. Once a child was free from soiling, he was instructed to go whenever he felt the sensation of rectal fullness (which had returned at this stage). No punishment was given for dirty pants nor any reward for clean ones. This operant procedure resulted in rapid elimination of encopresis in three of the four children.

Bach and Moylan (1975) treated a case of constipation and soiling in a six-year-old boy. The child also urinated inappropriately. He had been almost totally incontinent for two-and-a-half years, despite the efforts of two pediatricians and a psychiatrist. A daily regime of laxatives, suppositories, and/or enemas had been recommended by the physicians for this case of "functional megacolon." However, since the insertion of these agents and mandatory trips to the toilet were a great source of aversion to the parents and child, these programs were never consistently executed. The new behavioral program required the parents to give a money reward to the child since this had seemed to motivate him in the past. More specifically the boy was given 25¢ for every bowel movement in the toilet, 10¢ for every time he urinated in the commode, and 10¢ every morning that his bed was not wet. His parents were to give the money immediately and consistently after the desired behaviors occurred and to praise the child. They were instructed to ignore all inappropriate bowel and bladder movements, and to change the boy's clothes as perfunctorily as possible. After 12 weeks of this program it became apparent that the enuresis but not the encopresis was responding satisfactorily. On the premise that the boy had lost the sensation of rectal fullness due to chronic constipation, the parents were instructed to prompt the boy to defectate and to give him 5¢ for "just trying to go kaka." The later intervention produced marked improvement of the encopresis and the problem was eliminated after twenty weeks. A two-year follow-up revealed no recurrence of the soiling.

A normal five-year-old boy frequently soiled himself over a period of several months (Keehn, 1965). On psychological advice, the mother repeatedly told the child that whenever he emptied his bowel in the toilet she would give him a piece of chocolate. This procedure worked immediately and there was no sign of relapse two months after, when the frequency of chocolate reinforcement had been reduced to almost zero.

A long-standing problem of constipation in a three-year-old child was treated by Tomlinson (1970). The boy averaged only one movement a week although no soiling was present. When encouraged to eliminate the child reported that it was painful and, although willing to spend considerable time on the toilet, he said he had no elimination cues nor urge to defecate. Since the boy was capable of retaining feces for up to 10 days, chronic constipation was continually present and defecation was, indeed, likely to be painful. Medical examination, including barium X-rays revealed no physiological dysfunction. The diet changes recommended by several pediatricians were temporarily effective but usually for only a week following their introduction.

Treatment involved rewarding the boy with bubble gum following an adequate defecation. The boy was very fond of bubble gum and now could *only* obtain it by having a movement. He could have as many pieces of gum as he wanted for the remainder of that day, with the stipulation that he could not save any from one day to the next. The gum was displayed in the bathroom where it could be given immediately after a successful elimination. Verbal praise following the desired response was limited by the parents to a simple statement of "good." A mild laxative was administered daily for the first week of this program to increase the likelihood of defecation and to decrease the chances that it would be difficult or painful.

On the third day of this new procedure, voluntary defecation occurred. The rate of voluntary elimination then increased to five times per week for the next two weeks and then to six times per week where it remained for the next five months. Thus a chronic constipation problem was solved in a short time by giving the boy a powerful incentive.

Since birth, a four-year-old boy had been subjected to several hospitalizations, numerous inconclusive medical examinations, daily laxatives, and suppositories for chronic constipation. With the introduction of repetitive suggestions, laxatives, and a material reinforcer (popsicle for child and brother), bowel movements were accelerated from zero unless suppositories were used, to a rate of one per day without suppositories or laxatives of any kind. Suggestions consisted of holding the child after an involuntary elimination using a suppository, and saying in a hypnotic monotone, "You will soon be able to go potty by yourself every day; it will feel good, no more suppositories will be used. You will not have to go to the hospital anymore" (Perzan, Boulander, and Fischer, 1972).

An eight-year-old boy who had regressed to frequent encopresis at age seven was successfully treated by the use of concrete rewards for appropriate elimination during the school day. The boy was allowed to select his own rewards from a store and he chose small toy cars and a carrying case for them. Later he was given money or Green Stamps which he could trade for gifts from a catalog. Initially he was given a reward for each appropriate elimination, then, after about a week, he earned a reward only if he eliminated appropriately for an entire day. Soiling episodes were ignored by the adults, and he simply cleaned himself and changed his underwear (Young and Goldsmith, 1972). Other treatment efforts during the previous two years had failed, including psychotherapy for the child, and casework with the parents within a comprehensive therapeutic milieu.

Blechman (1978) treated five encopretic children by manipulating positive antecedents and consequences for appropriate toileting behavior, and did not use laxatives, prompting, or punishment. Each child was referred by a pediatrician after medical tests had ruled out Hirchsprung's disease. Laxatives and diet prescribed by the pediatrician had been unsuccessful, although the colons of the children had all been cleaned out. The first step in treatment involved asking the parents to check their child's pants three times a day and record any sign of soiling; they also recorded each bowel movement in the toilet. The parents provided the child with a reward (a favorite food e.g., bubble gum, or activity e.g., playtime with Daddy) immediately after they observed appropriate toileting behavior (clean pants; bowel movement in the toilet). The child was made responsible for cleaning his or her own body and clothes after soiling. Special toys and books that particularly appealed to the child were purchased and reserved for use only when the child sat on the toilet. The child's successes were recorded on a chart in the bathroom. The parents were told to praise successes and to be nonchalant about the absence of success. They were advised to expect gradual success.

The results revealed that rewarding clean pants alone was less effective than a combined reward for bowel movements in the toilet and clean pants. One reason for this seems to be that stool retention and chronic constipation precede the soiling of most encopretic children. As a result, the bowel movement reward acts on the earliest link in the chain of desirable, substitute behaviors—the deliberate effort to expel feces in the toilet. Altering the toilet setting ambiance by providing toys and books also seemed to contribute to successful treatment of the five cases. The toys may have diverted the child's attention from the physical pain of elimination; or, they may have lowered the unpleasantness of the bathroom (a place where the encopretic child is forced to spend a lot of unproductive time).

Penalties

Ferinden and Van Handel (1970) present the case of George, a seven-year-old boy diagnosed as emotionally immature and having psychogenic megacolon (dilation of the colon) with a five-year history of soiling and chronic constipation. George was referred to the school psychologist because he soiled almost daily and sometimes as often as three times in a school day. After each mishap, George had been sent home to be cleaned up and obtain fresh clothing.

The following punishment procedure was implemented. George was not only required to bring a change of clothing to school, but also to clean himself and wash his soiled clothes in cold water with a mildly abrasive soap. In addition, he had to make up time lost from the classroom after school hours.

Simultaneously, George met with the psychologist to discuss the social implications of his behavior. In one of these sessions, he admitted that he was acting like a baby because he would like to stay home all the time with his mother and watch television.

The aversive procedure produced a marked reduction in the incidence of classroom soiling and George soiled himself only nine more times after the procedure was initiated. In addition to the elimination of soiling in school and at home (no relapse after six months), the boy also showed more positive peer relationships.

A noted pediatrician, Edward Henoch, reported success with encopretic children by injecting one or two doses of ergotin or distilled water into the child's rectum. A few smart strokes on the child's bottom immediately after the injection were found to considerably enhance the effect of this treatment (Henoch, 1889).

PSYCHOANALYTIC APPROACH

Psychoanalytic theorists view disorders such as encopresis to result from unconscious, repressed conflicts in the child. Conflicts develop early when the child's demands for gratification of sexual and aggressive impulses meet with parental demands for conformity to their own standards of behavior. Parental demands to control the pleasurable act of defecation, for example, are believed to result in tension or anxiety. This anxiety is translated into visible signs of disturbance—such as soiling.

The basic treatment strategy of the psychoanalytic approach has been the resolution of the conflict causing the anxiety. Methods of anxiety reduction include interpretations to facilitate insight, and cathartic acting-out of aggression through play therapy (Sachs, 1974). None of these therapeutic methods treat the symtoms, since they are not viewed as the root cause but only outward signs of the underlying conflict. According to psychodynamic formulation, underlying conflicts resulting in fecal soiling range from fear of castration (Sterba, 1949; Ross, 1953) and coercive toilet training (Huschka, 1942); to hostility towards parents (Pinkerton, 1958).

The first article by an analyst dealing solely with encopresis was by Lehman (1944). He observed that the term "encopresis" was first used in 1926 by Weissenberg who regarded fecal incontinence as etiologically analogous to enuresis, that is, both are psychogenic in origin. Lehman reviewed the psychiatric and psychoanalytic literature and described the psychotherapy of four cases, emphasizing the need for parental love, especially from the mother, if the child is to establish effective control over the bowels. In his psychotherapeutic approach he focused less on the transference than on making unconscious fantasies conscious. In addition, he helped the parents to be either less compulsively demanding, or more lovingly attentive to these children. The soiling decreased as a result of the diminished environmental stresses and as they gained an intellectual understanding of their preverbal expression of conflicts.

Warson *et al.* (1954) presented a case study involving a six-year-old girl who exhibited an encopresis problem since infancy. She was the second of three children. Her upper-middle-class parents were highly intellectual, compulsive persons who revealed little warmth. They were disgusted with her soiling and emphasized the need for their child to conform and show normal cleanliness. The mother was preoccupied with feelings of inadequacy and failure as a parent.

When the child was two, her older brother required hospitalization and extended home care because of an illness; at the same time, her father was transferred to another city, so that the family had to move. During this hectic period, the child received little parental attention and changed from a happy child to a whiny, fearful, demanding one. At age three, the child strained to avoid bowel movements and began almost continuous fecal soiling. She seemed indifferent to the problem and refused to cooperate with her mother, who spent a great deal of time keeping her clean. No physical basis for the problem was discovered. The child and her mother were seen in parallel treatment sessions over the course of a year.

The child was seen in a permissive form of play therapy for 42 sessions over the period of 14 months. During the initial sessions, her compulsive, critical traits were evident in her calling toys "dirty," "black," "nasty brown," or "broken." After touching any of these condemned items, she would run to the playroom sink to wash her hands. Her critical comments then switched to her siblings and she began to attack them verbally or by smearing with finger paints. Although she seemed excited and delighted with finger painting, she would quickly become anxious and rush to scrub her hands. Gradually she was able to spend a whole hour pushing a "brother doll" through a mound of brown finger paint. Next, mother dolls, who were viewed as being angry and punishing, were rubbed with sand and water in a hostile manner. In a later session, the child expressed verbal anger toward her mother for the first time and then became very frightened about it. In subsequent sessions, she became more spontaneous about verbalizing such feelings as fears about being sent away from home; her panic on one occasion in early childhood when she had flushed the toilet and it had overflowed; and hostile-competitive feelings toward her siblings and mother. She also began enjoying making messes with clay and finger paints. She remarked, for example, how wonderful the "soft, squishy mud" felt. The patient then began having the dolls make bowel movements with clay and finger paints. She talked about some mothers who did not want their children ever to have bowel movements. After asking the therapist to clean up the mess made by the dolls, she seemed to relax when it was done in a matter-of-fact manner. The child seemed to receive a "corrective emotional experience" from the therapist (See Anna Freud 1965, p. 231), who was seen as a "new object." During the final sessions, she began playing in a constructive fashion with the paints and expressed the desire to terminate therapy because she was not soiling anymore.

In separate sessions, the child's mother was able to express pent-up feelings of inadequacy, resentment, and hostility toward both her husband and mother. She was helped to see that her own mother raised her in a strict, perfectionistic, overly controlled way, just as she was raising her own daughter. With a great deal of acceptance, understanding, and support, the mother seemed to gain more confidence in herself as a parent.

Follow-ups 2 and 12 months after the termination of therapy revealed that the child remained free of symptoms and she was described as a "changed" child. Both she and her mother seemed happy, friendly, and more self-confident.

Segall (1957) treated a two-year-old girl who would retain her feces for several days and then empty her bowels only in bed. Other disturbances included feeding difficulty, stubbornness, fear of dirt, and enuresis. Although the child was never fully trained, she did not experience difficulty with defecation until six months prior to the referral. At this time she seemed to suffer a trauma in that her parents left her for a time with a maternal aunt. Feeling deprived, the child seemed to regress to more infantile behavior (including soiling) which she associated with parental love and attention. Her soiling also seemed to be an act of rebellion against her compulsively clean mother.

In play therapy the child showed obvious delight in smearing water and sand and calling it the "therapist's kaka." The therapist verbalized this pleasure for the child, and reassured the child it was all right to have dirty hands. In contrast to the mother who seemed overconcerned with cleanliness, the therapist remained calm and accepting towards the child's water and sand play. After two play sessions the child for the first time asked for the pot at home and made her bowel movements into it. In her play she seemed to work through her anxieties over dirt and toileting functioning. The child seemed to obtain symbolic satisfaction from her play which she felt had been denied to her. Sterba (1949) described a similar case of a boy, who after having established a relationship with her, quickly gave up withholding his feces. After six play sessions the child did not soil again at home, although he did continue to show some anal agressiveness such as obstinacy and stubbornness.

Call *et al.* (1963) found that the primary symptom in children with psychogenic megacolon is that of withholding bowel movement. They noted three primary factors in the etiology of this fecal holding: (1) failure of the parents to provide an adequate relational basis in which a meaningful pattern of communication with the outside world can develop; (2) erotization of the anal and bowel functions in an infant due to excessive parental interest in the child's anus and bowel functioning; and (3) traumatic events related to the use of the toilet and the bathroom. The authors recommend therapy for the parents which provides them with a supportive climate while they give up their overconcern with the child's anal functioning, helps them to understand the child's current struggles, and assists them in their efforts to help the child resolve oedipal problems by identifying with the same sex parent.

Finally, Shane (1967) reports the case of Stevie, a nine-year-old boy, who had been encopretic and enuretic almost all his life. He was seen four times a week by the analyst, his mother was seen every other week, and his father occasionally. In therapy, he exhibited sudden and unpredictable aggressive outbursts. Like his mother, he would be warm and affectionate one minute and hostile the next. Therapeutic techniques included putting into words his angry feelings (such as the desire to get even with his mother for preoedipal frustrations by soiling); interpreting his wish to be protected and loved—especially by his mother; encouragement of identification with the therapist (as a source of external control), and working through of castration anxieties. After two years of analysis, the encopresis and enuresis ceased, although he continued treatment for over three years for his continued impulsiveness which the author has found to be associated with encopresis through adulthood. A step-by-step progression through the developmental lines (from wetting and soiling to bladder and bowel control) outlined by Anna Freud was noted in this case.

FAMILY THERAPY AND COUNSELING APPROACHES

The main difference between the individual approaches previously described, and a family approach is a shift of emphasis in therapy from individual behavior to family interactions and relational systems. A major assumption of this approach is that maladaptive interaction patterns within the family play a significant role in the origins and maintenance of the encopresis problem. Family therapy would seem indicated, for example, when a child hostilely expels his feces as a way of getting back at his parents. Also, when a child is soiling because of faulty toilet training, family counseling as to effective toileting practices seems indicated. In both cases the parents are assumed to play a role in the problem and, thus, are involved in treatment.

A variety of maladaptive parental attitudes, traits, and childrearing practices have been reported to be connected with childhood encopresis. In one study, families of encopretic children were found to exhibit the following behaviors: the withholding of vital information, an aspect of the relationship, or of tangible things from the child; the tendency to infantilize the child; the presence of anger and its denial; and a general distortion of communication (Baird, 1974). Therefore the correction of the dysfunctional family patterns should be the first step in the child's treatment.

Anthony (1957) distinguishes between two types of encopretic children. The "continuous" (never had control) child is a dirty child coming from a dirty family, burdened with every conceivable sort of social problem. Much external pressure is needed before the mother will agree to treatment. This child does not need psychotherapy, but rather consistent habit training administered by a warm, interested person. By identifying with a normal adult he can develop some degree of disgust for the symptom. He can be reasonably stabilized in a period of three to five months. The "discontinuous" (had control but lost it) child, on the other hand, is the compulsive child of a compulsive family. He is overcontrolled and inhibited in his emotional life and scrupulous in his habits. He is very defensive about his symptom and difficult to treat. He tends to be a deeply disturbed child who needs prolonged psychotherapy and some measure of protection from his mother and their sadomasochistic relationship. A disappearance of an exaggerated disgust reaction is the first hopeful therapeutic sign. In family therapy the parents need to learn to be more accepting and easygoing as opposed to domineering and perfectionistic.

Perfectionistic parents who set high standards for themselves and their family have also been associated with encopresis in certain children by Plachetta (1976). Often these parents are very religious and run the household in a strict fashion. Parental expectations of orderliness, cleanliness, and performance are evident. Often, one or more of these parents is nervous, highstrung and always in a hurry. Such parents can benefit from short-term counseling as to ways to reduce tension and pressure on children.

After an intensive study of the families of 10 encopretic boys (ages 7 to 13), Hoag *et al.* (1971) report that none of the children had been successfully breast-fed and none was the favorite child within the family constellation. The boys expressed denigrated self concepts. They felt unloved and unwanted but were unable to express any resentment. They were lonely, depressed, dependent boys who denied their symptoms and yearned for acceptance. Their mothers were compulsive, frequently depressed women who felt frustrated in both marital and maternal roles. They were emotionally unavailable to their sons yet represented the only source of primary nurturance and affection. The mother-child relationship was characterized by maternal ambivalence, alternating between excessive rigidity and permissiveness. Beneath a critical and perfectionistic exterior, the fathers were passively detached and emotionally distant. The children were seen in play therapy for about 15 sessions while their parents attended weekly group sessions. Half of the children (mostly secondary soilers) showed considerable improvement. Successful treatment was highly correlated with the outcome of parental treatment, that is, the ability of the parents to relate the soiling to family functioning, rather than exclusively to the child.

Bemporad *et al.* (1971) also found that 14 of 17 encopretic children (ages 5 to 13) showed a similarity of character structure and family background. Physically they were all small, pale boys who had a distinctively sick look. They showed a lack of maturity and an excessive dependence on their mothers for their own sense of values. Beneath their passive and benign facades, however, they exhibited a good deal of anger. During clinical interviews they rarely volunteered information and remained guarded and sullen. Eleven of the 14 had been trained prior to 18 months of age, and the training had been reported to be difficult, coercive or prolonged.

The parents of eight of these children had been divorced, while the fathers of the remaining six were either completely or frequently absent from the home. The fathers were passive, depressed and isolated people who seemed to be intimidated by their domineering wives and to react either in a petulant, hostile manner or by dissociating themselves from the family. In contrast, the mothers were characteristically domineering and overly involved in the children's everyday life. They seemed to vacillate between overbearing intrusion into the life of the child and a rejecting, excluding type of behavior. This inconsistency in their relationships with their children seemed to be a reflection of a more basic ambivalence toward their own role in life, that is, submissive vs. aggressive. Seven of the 14 mothers seemed clinically depressed.

According to Bemporad, the encopretic children seem to use soiling as a hostile and attention-getting maneuver in the course of a hostile-dependent relationship with their mothers and within the context of the absence of the father. In six of the boys the encopresis rapidly ceased or abated when their fathers returned home or when they were induced, through therapy, to spend more time with their sons. In another child, the soiling stopped when the mother remarried.

Sometimes when a child is helped to stop soiling he starts displaying outbursts of aggressive behavior at home, such as temper tantrums and cursing. Usually this aggressiveness is not a new symptom that has been substituted for the old. Indeed, these children tend to have thrown temper tantrums earlier in life and the encopresis seems to have substituted for the violent outbursts (Balson, 1973; Young and Goldsmith, 1972). In these cases the child needs instruction as to more acceptable ways of expressing anger and coping with frustration. In addition, the parents often need counseling in ways of coping with temper outbursts by the child.

Andolfi (1978) used Minuchin's "structural family therapy" approach to treat an encopretic child. The basic goal of this therapy is to change the family structure rather than just to offer guidance so as to relieve the presenting problem. The individual disorder is used as a point of entry to observe and change the family's interaction patterns, functional and dysfunctional communication channels, personal and interpersonal boundaries, and resistances to change. The author presents a case study of Andy—a 12-year-old boy who had been "crapping in his pants" several times a day, even at school. After negative results from lab tests at a hospital the child was referred for brief family therapy by the pediatrician.

Family history revealed that the parents had been separated for several years and the father was living with another woman and kept only sporadic contacts with the mother and other three children—Sandra 13, Charlene 7, and Robert 6. The mother worked as a cleaning lady and took pride in her role as a mother and provider. Quite self-sufficient, the children assumed many responsibilities while the mother was at work.

The first point of entry into the family was to discuss the encopresis problem in detail, and to assess the motivation of the family members to help resolve the problem. The mother was worried that the soiling represented a "mental problem" related to her husband's hospitalization in the past for psychiatric reasons. The boy seemed ashamed of his incontinence since it was not suitable to his age.

Since the mother was typically too busy to play with her children, the initial therapeutic approach was to arrange play sessions for the mother and the four children. From these sessions it was evident that the two older children formed one subgroup, the younger sibs another. The encopresis had confused this hierarchy since Andy had regressed to the younger group. The therapist attempted to form an alliance with Andy by asking him for the meaning of some black slang expressions. The boy was pleased and proud of his role as a consultant. The therapist also restructured the family interactions by making Andy's and his older sister's chores more equal at home (his sister had been assuming greater responsibilities and Andy had resented this). Both these restructuring tasks gave Andy a sense of greater competence and reduced the parental role played by Sandra which enabled her to function more as an adolescent.

At this point in therapy the therapist formed an exclusive alliance with Andy in that he offered to have private talks with him to help him solve his encopresis. The boy readily agreed to this, and to the task of keeping a personal diary in which he noted when and how he soiled his pants each day. This alliance changed the *relational meaning of the symptom* since Andy was now acting out for the therapist, rather than for his family. The encopresis, which initially was a means of communication within the family, became the central content of a growing relationship between the boy and the therapist. At the same time, talking about the incontinence as if it were a work task, with schedules and deadlines, ultimately rendered it ridiculous and untenable. By this *strategy of provocation* a therapist directly challenges the disorder while simultaneously making an effort to enhance the person by encouraging and reinforcing positive aspects of his behavior.

The therapist's alliance with Andy and the provocative strategy represented only part of a broader plan which had at first required a redefinition of boundaries and responsibilities at the level of the sibling subsystem and then at the level of the parents. Since the parents were separated, this second task had to focus on the mother via individual therapy sessions. In these sessions the mother reported improvement in the encopresis and no longer even mentioned the problem. Rather she seemed to seek help for her own conflicts, particularly relating to a man who had been providing her with affection and support, but who also brought guilt to her since she feared the children would blame her for not dedicating herself to them. The therapist not only helped her resolve this conflict but also suggested that she be more open with the children in discussing their father. In a subsequent family session the children openly discussed their father and their anxious and confused feelings about his hospitalization and why he did not come to visit them.

In another session with the mother the therapist discussed the possibility of the father forming a more positive and active relationship with the children. Such a move would make it easier for the mother to accept her relationship with another man without feeling guilty. The mother agreed to this and Andy was selected as the most suitable person to contact the father. The father accepted Andy's invitation to attend the next family session. At this session the father seemed very affectionate with the children although embarrassed about his long absence. Several more family sessions were devoted to negotiating new ways for the father and children to form closer affective bonds. In the last session with just the parents present, the therapist supported the father's efforts to be closer to the children, notwithstanding the mother's doubts that he would sustain this commitment.

A two-year follow-up revealed that the father had maintained his contact with the children, and was very happy about the weekly visits by Andy whom he was teaching to repair cars. The mother had found a less tiring job and was continuing her extramarital relationship, which no longer caused her to feel guilty towards her children.

Sheinbein (1975) strongly asserts that both the encopretic child and his family should be included in the treatment plan. Thus, he advocates a novel triadic approach that combines behavior modification principles with conjoint family therapy. Before treatment, of course, neurological causes, such as Hirschsprung's disease, must be ruled out. (Hirschsprung's disease is a primarily neurological disorder where the colon is unable to respond to pressure with the appropriate defecation reflex.)

In the triadic behavioral approach, the therapist first provides the family with a positive reinforcement procedure that gives the child material and/or social rewards for appropriate defecation. The child is made an ally in the process and encouraged to be responsible for its success. The parents are involved in this procedure as monitors and reinforcers. The child no longer fears the parents, as he knows exactly what to expect and feels that it is up to him now.

Once the encopresis problem is under control and the family members are able to relax, the therapist seeks to resolve the underlying causes of the symptom by conjoint family sessions. Typically, the parents are compulsive, overly intellectualizing people who isolate feelings and have trouble becoming close to one another. The therapist therefore encourages the family members to be more honest and open with each other by disclosing feelings and making clear, direct statements of needs and wishes. Through this process they reveal their individuality and become more lovable to one another. It is important that the therapist serve as a model for giving support, for negotiating, and for providing firm, consistent limits. He must also demonstrate confidence that the treatment will work. The family will attempt to undermine his efforts by diverse strategies, including a proclivity to complain rather than to solve problems, but the therapist should not be put off. The parent-child-therapist triad must continue to struggle to overcome interpersonal distance and misunderstanding.

In the triadic behavioral approach, advocated by Sheinbein, the therapist seeks to change the family interaction patterns as well as the child. The basic premise is that if the goals of open and honest communication among family members are achieved, then deviant behaviors become unnecessary and disappear. The theory is based on the triad-based family therapy approach of G. H. Zuk.

Until recently, family therapy has not been reported to be a particularly effective remedy for encopresis (Halpern, 1977), although there have been numerous articles dealing with the encopretic child and his family. It has been suggested that if the soiling is to be the exclusive concern of the parents, it will have to be quickly brought under control if the family is to continue in therapy. It would seem, then, that the optimal strategy would be to bring the encopresis quickly under control by the use of cathartics and operant conditioning, and then use this initial success to motivate the family to work on deeper, more complex problems by means of family therapy.

COMPREHENSIVE APPROACHES

Believing that encopresis occurs as a result of a complex interaction of organic and psychological factors, an increasing number of therapists are recommending a multifaceted approach which simultaneously treats a wide range of systems (organic, behavioral, cognitive and environmental) so as to achieve the most efficacious results.

Rather than stressing a single strategy, core construct, or critical mode of functioning, the comprehensive or multimodal approach (Lazarus, 1976) asserts that a variety of specific techniques should be used in accord with the needs of the specific case . This multimodal approach supplies a framework and organizing rationale for applying technical eclecticism. Also, combined treatment methods have been found to maximize the probability of sustained remission of disorders such as encopresis (Wright and Bunch, 1977).

Based upon his extensive experience in treating encopretic children within a hospital setting, Wright (1973) recommends a standardized treatment program which stresses both physiological and behavioral intervention. Prior to treatment, a comprehensive diagnostic assessment should be made which includes both medical and psychological information. A medical exam should indicate whether the disorder has a physical etiology (Hirschsprung's disease or obstruction), if megacolon is present, information about the muscle tone of the colon, and the characteristics of the stools (hard vs. soft; large vs. small).

A psychological interview should ascertain: (1) whether the child ever achieved bowel training; (2) age continence was lost; (3) if coercive toilet training practices were present; (4) whether there is a history of stomach pains or gastrointestinal (GI) problems; (5) psychological problems other than soiling; (6) events that seem to lead up to or coincide with soiling; (7) nature of previous attempts by parents and/or therapists to eliminate the problem; (8) list of rewards that child will work for; (9) family history of bowel or GI difficulties; (10) if psychological factors seem to be a causative factor in the soiling, do these factors still exist?; (11) child-rearing strategies employed by parents that may be deleterious; and (12) any fear of the toilet due to previous trauma or pain.

The first step in treatment involves "selling" the parents on the efficacy of conditioning methods, to establish in them the expectation that treatment will be successful. The parents are warned that lack of consistency in strictly following the conditioning program is a common cause of failure. Consistency is defined as something that happens 100 percent of the time; 90 percent consistency is seen as no better than 10 percent. To promote consistency, daily written records and at least weekly check-ins with the therapist are required.

Next, three reinforcers (two positive and one negative) are identified for the conditioning program. The most common positive reinforcer, in Wright's experience, has been the opportunity to earn time alone with parents, during which period the child determines the nature of the activity, such as playing a game, going for a ride.

Other rewards include tokens for purchase of toys or candy, toys themselves, trips, and tickets to movies. Negative reinforcers include such consequences as 30 minutes in the bathtub, extra chores, sitting in a chair for 15 minutes, and loss of free play time. Any incidence of defecation in the toilet is then positively reinforced, as is going for one day without soiling. A punishment is administered after each soiling episode.

The child is told he must try to defecate on arising in the morning. If he cannot produce at least ¼ to ½ cup of feces on his own, he is given a glycerine suppository (no prescription needed) and allowed to eat breakfast. By the end of breakfast, the child will usually need to defecate. If not, he is given a Fleet enema before going to school. This absolute predictability of defecation at a fixed time is considered essential to treatment. The daily defecation also allows the child's colon to regain its normal shape and muscle tone and prevents soiling.

At a specified time (after school, after supper, or shortly before bedtime) the child's clothing is examined. When there is no soiling, he receives a reward. When there is soiling, he receives a mild punishment described earlier.

The final and most difficult step of the program involves weaning the child from the suppositories after daily bowel movements are established for two weeks and soiling discontinued. Initially, one day of the week is chosen, and all external aids to defecation are eliminated for that day. With each additional week without soiling, another day's cathartics (external aids) are discontinued. If soiling occurs during the weaning process, one day's cathartics are added for each soiling episode until the child is receiving cathartics every day or until he again goes a week without soiling. At this point, the weaning process begins anew. If a child goes two weeks without soiling after all cathartics are discontinued, the program is terminated.

Wright reports that the program has generally been effective in alleviating encopresis in an average of 15 to 20 weeks. Sometimes parent counseling and/or family therapy is added to the program if it seems warranted and the parents are agreeable.

This program, which can be administered by parents at home, seems to offer a practical, economical, and efficient means of treating the encopretic child. As in any home management program the parent's ability to follow the routine rigorously is a crucial aspect of successful treatment. Logan reports success with this program for both primary and secondary encopresis. Other therapists (Schaefer, 1978) have employed Wright's standardized program and reported equally positive results.

The management program advocated by Wright is relatively simple to explain to parents and can be readily supervised. According to Wright and Walker (1977) it places a major responsibility on the child, less on the parents, and only a supervisory role for the therapist or pediatrician. It is very important for the success of this program that the rewards be ones which the child finds very attractive, while the punishments be ones he definitely wants to avoid. Children who relapse after having successfully completed the program generally respond quite well to the same program again, which generally takes less time than the first.

Young (1973) recommends a treatment which capitalizes on the natural physiology of the GI tract. Mass movements of the colon occur usually after a meal or fluid intake because of increased colonic motor activity (gastrocolonic reflex) and hyperactive terminal ileum (gastroileal reflex). The location of the ileum is presented in Figure 2. Mass movements of the colon empty the contents of the proximal colon into the more distal sections, and frequently these movements result in an increased urge to defecate. It takes about 20 to 30 minutes after ingesting food or drink for the colonic sensation to occur, and the most common time for the reflex to appear is during the first hour after arising in the morning. Accumulated feces in the rectum are removed before treating an encopretic child, to increase perception of the reflexes. After a child awakens in the morning, his parents give him or her a warm drink or food. After 20 to 30 minutes, the child is taken to the toilet and the parents suggest bowel action. The child is allowed to sit on the toilet for no more than 10 minutes. If successful, he is given approval; if not, a nonchalant attitude is shown. This procedure is repeated at the other meals, if possible. To relieve colonic inertia and assist the gastroileal reflex, most of the 24 children in this study were given Senokot (one-half to two tablets) before going to bed at night. If fecal impaction was present it was removed by an enema. The results indicated that 19 children were successfully treated within 12 months, three were successful in over 12 months, and two children did not respond. During follow-up, four children suffered relapses that were successfully treated by repeating the procedure.

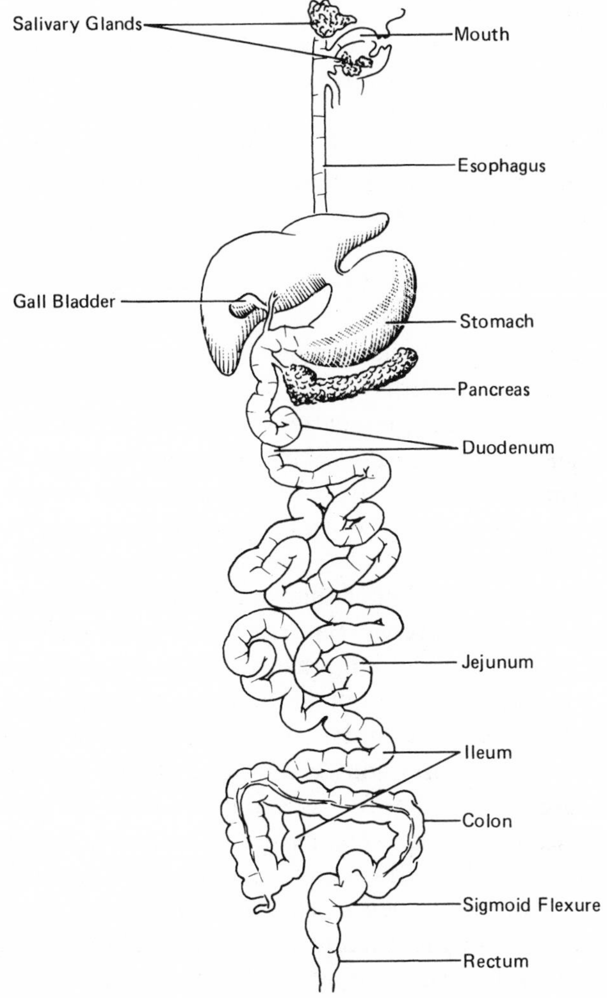

Figure 2. The Human Digestive System.

Lambley (1976) treated a 12-year-old orphan who had been complaining of encopresis for the past three years. Previous treatment had consisted of psychoanalysis, play therapy, and behavior modification. A five-phase treatment plan was put into effect:

1. The therapist spent a number of beginning sessions forming a relationship and establishing trust.

2. The boy was placed on a nonirritating diet.
3. The boy was asked to see the therapist whenever he felt stomach pain (due to constipation), and this distraction usually ensured proper defecation.
4. The boy was asked to relate all feelings of hostility towards others to the therapist, who would then try to intervene with others to resolve the conflict.
5. Once soiling had been eliminated the therapist found other staff members to handle his functions.

Daily monitoring of the soiling revealed that the program was successful after two months.

Apart from relapses after eating things like dried fruit, the boy showed no major relapse in soiling after nine months. The author attributes this success to the comprehensiveness of the treatment which involved cognitive, organic, behavioral and environmental systems.

Based upon a similar belief that one technique will not suffice in the therapy of encopresis, Halpern (1977) advocates an eclectic approach. After ascertaining that there is no physical cause, the therapist asks the child to mention items of value to him or her which can be used as rewards. The physiology of the GI tract is explained to the parents and to the older child. Dulcolax suppositories are used once a day for three days because they are quick acting (usually produce a movement within a half hour), are less aversive than enemas, and give the child an immediate success experience which can be promptly rewarded. The author has found that this combination of organic therapy and behavior modification brings quick success for most encopretic children. For the few children who show intense fears of toileting, systematic desensitization of the fears by the parents is indicated. For those children who never achieved continence, a supportive program which rewards appropriate use of the toilet is advised. In those cases where the child tends to form hard stools which are expelled with discomfort, a stool softener such as doctylsodium (colace) is added to the program.

Finally, Wright and Bunch (1977) reported success with a three-year-old girl who had chronic constipation, by using a combination of behavioral intervention and physiological treatment. Behavioral intervention consisted of the following:

1. The child was asked to choose five to 10 small toys and candies to be used as reinforcers. These items, replenished weekly, were placed on a shelf just out of reach but visible.
2. When the child requested aid in using the toilet, her parents immediately took her to the toilet, but said nothing unless the child had a movement.
3. For each BM the child was immediately praised and given her choice of a small toy or candy. These reinforcers were gradually withdrawn, contingent upon weekly progress.
4. The therapist monitored the program by weekly telephone calls and monthly clinic visits.

Medical intervention consisted of 3 teaspoons of mineral oil (MO) per day, so as to elicit BM's consistently. When BM's were occurring at a consistent frequency (greater than twice the pretreatment frequency for 18 days), the dosage was reduced to 2 teaspoons per day. After the BM's had stabilized, the laxative dosage was reduced to 1 teaspoon per day, then ½ teaspoon, and finally it was discontinued. When a recurrence of BM infrequency was observed, the laxative dosage was temporarily strengthened to the previous level. If this change in medical intervention did not relieve the symptom relapse, a parallel change was made in the behavioral intervention. By week 12 of this program the child was having eight movements per week and no relapse was found at 39-, 67-, and 93-week follow-ups.

Keat (1976) applied Lazarus's multimodal approach in counseling a nine-year-old girl with encopresis and other difficulties. The child would usually hide per pants after soiling, and the odor in her room would become unbearable after a few days. After a comprehensive review of the possible modes of intervention (Behavior, Affect, Sensation, Imagery, Cognition, Interpersonal Relationships and Drugs-Diet, it was decided to employ two direct techniques for the encopresis: Behavioral Contact and Restitution). The parents and child were helped to make a contract regarding the encopresis, i.e., specific rewards for periods of no soiling, which was posted on the refrigerator. By "restitution" the child was required to clean up her "accidents" and wash out her clothing. After two months the soiling ceased. Noteworthy is the fact that other techniques were employed to teach the child effective ways to deal with her anger, which reduced the child's need to get back at her mother by soiling.

A successful pediatric program based on dietary control, bowel training, and family counseling is described by Hein and Beerends (1978). In treating 18 cases of functional encopresis, the authors first counseled the parents that the child did not have voluntary control over the bowel, and that the goal of the procedure was to carry out bowel training using normal physiologic factors such as diet and regular use of the commode. The importance of having the child's feet placed firmly on the floor or a similar surface was stressed and many parents were instructed to build a small platform around the base of the adult toilet for these children. While avoiding punishment and punitive attitudes, the parents were to inform the child that the program was important, had worked for many other children, and might work for them also.

An instruction sheet given the parents advised them as follows: (1) have the child sit on the stool/potty 10 minutes after each meal; (2) give the child a Fleet enema the first evening of the program and another the following morning; (3) limit the child's ingestion of bananas, apples and milk (16 ounces per day only), while encouraging the child to eat bran cereal, vegetables (spinach, lettuce, cabbage, corn), drink extra water, and once a day for the first week have either 2 ounces of prune juice or three to five stewed prunes. Milk of magnesia was added when the diet alone did not improve the consistency of the stool. Assured that following the instructions carefully would give an excellent chance of success, the parents returned for monthly follow-up visits. Within an average of one to two months of treatment (one child required six months), 14 of the 18 children had stopped soiling completely. Although many of the children had emotional problems, the authors concluded that the soiling itself perpetuated much of the child's current problem so that a psychiatric referral was not needed. The value of supportive counseling for the family and understanding the gastroileal reflex (Young, 1973) is stressed in this study.

In a large medical center, Levine and Bakow (1976) initiated a pediatric treatment program for 127 children with encopresis. Any child over four who regularly passed stools (formed, semiformed, or liquid) into his or her underwear or pajamas was considered to have encopresis. A history of significant constipation in infancy was reported in 33 percent of the cases, and parents described difficulty in toilet-training 45 percent of the children. The first step in treatment involved a careful history-taking to ascertain the etiology, manifestations and complications of each child's encopresis. A plain X-ray film of the abdomen was also taken to determine the degree of stool retention. Barium enemas and rectal biopsies were not taken unless there were clear signs of Hirschsprung's neurological disorder. During the first counseling session, the child and parents received counseling concerning the problem. A unique characteristic of encopretic children is that they tend not to know of any other children with the same disorder. Thus, the child and parents are informed that many other youngsters suffer from this problem. After giving the family an opportunity to express their feelings about the disorder they were reassured that no one was perceived to be at fault or was to be accused of causing it. A major goal of this initial interview was to alleviate guilt and shame, and enable the family to talk openly about the problem in a supportive environment.

It was found that many of the children harbored a mystical concept about their bowels since they had been told by other professionals that the problem would vanish when they were "ready" to have it do so, or that they were soiling to get attention. This tended to create confusion and an aura of magic about the symptom. A history of inconsistent parental management and conflicting professional advice tended to complicate the problem. To "demystify" the disorder, the pediatricians in this study discussed normal intestinal function in a simple way during the first visit. They drew a cross-section of a normal colon, showing the walls made of muscle and the central lumen within that muscle, through which waste passes. The child was told that children tended to hold in their waste for a variety of reasons, such as fear of the toilet, discomfort in moving their bowels, or because they were too busy playing. A second diagram was then drawn for each child showing an intestine that had become blocked up with large amounts of waste material and had been so distended that its muscles were thin and weak. It was explained that his or her problem involved such muscles that had been stretched and were weakened. The basic theme of treatment was the development of muscle tone. This was linked to concepts of autonomy, independence, effectiveness, control, and growing up. The child's treatment program was compared to a training program for an athlete, with assurance that consistent effort by the child would result in muscle build-up in the intestines and marked improvement in bowel control. In light of the above it was explained to the family that it was not really the child's fault he or she was having "accidents." In addition to the weak muscles, it was pointed out that the distended colon was less sensitive to pressure and thus offered less of a warning to children as to the need to defecate. It was also suggested that the child had become so accustomed to fecal odor as to lose awareness of when soiling occurred. Almost invariably, the family showed relief and cooperation when this positive, nonaccusatory approach was used.

No punishment or negative comments were used during the program. Where the mother seemed overinvolved, an effort was made to transfer accountability to the child and physician. Mothers were urged to avoid regular contact with the child's anogenital area and the child was encouraged to clean his own body. Underwear was to be washed by the mother to avoid any suggestion of parental retribution.

The first physiological phase of treatment involved the use of bowel cathartics, that is, enemas and laxatives. It was explained that this was needed for muscle training. Home management was organized around treatment cycles, each lasting three days. On the first day of the three-day cycle, the child was given two adult hyperphosphate enemas (Fleet's) in succession. On the second day of each cycle the child was given a biscodyl (Dulcolax) suppository right after school and again early in the evening. On the third day, the child was administered a 10-mg biscodyl tablet right after school and one in the evening. Three or four consecutive cycles were used for each child, followed by a repeat X-ray film of the abdomen to document changes and determine if further cycles were needed. In mild cases and in children under seven, one half of the above doses was used in each cycle.

For those cases of particularly severe obstipation (blockage) or where there were psychological or social reasons for avoiding enemas at home, children were admitted to the hospital where they were given high-normal saline enemas (approximately 750 cc two or three times per day for a seven-year-old child). Moreover, they received biscodyl suppositories twice each day and were encouraged to use the toilet at specified times.

The initial bowel evacuation phase was not considered complete until an X-ray film showed evidence of little, if any, retained feces.

This was thought essential because often after enemas had produced high yields and the child's abdomen was found to be soft to the touch, X-ray films had revealed abundant retained stool. Rapid relapses are common if a child's bowels are not completely disimpacted.

After a well-cleaned-out bowel was documented, the maintenance phase of the program was implemented. For most of the children, this involved the use of light mineral oil at an average initial dose (for a seven-year-old) of 30 cc twice each day. This dose was quickly raised in those children who did not have regular bowel movements at least once every two days. The family had been informed in advance that the light mineral oil would have to be taken for at least six months. The mineral oil was then tapered gradually in successful cases. While receiving mineral oil, the children were encouraged to take two multiple vitamin pills per day between oil dosages to minimize possible effects of malabsorption of fat-soluble vitamins.

In addition, the parents and child were instructed to look for early evidence of recurring stool retention, such as larger-caliber stools, less frequent defecation, abdominal pain, reappearance of soiling, or excessive leakage of mineral oil. When such signs were noted, the child was given a supplemental oral laxative for one or two weeks. Senna concentrate (Senokot) or danthron (Mondane) were used for this purpose. The Senna was given in a dose of one tablet or 5.0 cc of the syrup extract daily. Danthron was given at a starting dose of 37.5 mg. The senna preparation was utilized first and, if necessary, the dose was increased. If abdominal pains occurred or if the senna was not effective, danthron was given up to a dose of 75 mg. The parents were urged strongly never to use suppositories or enemas for relapses, since the emphasis after the initial catharsis was to avoid recurrent direct "anal assaults."

A third component of the program involved helping the child feel comfortable on a toilet. The children were told that this was a critical part of their "muscle training," and that they needed to sit on the toilet with adequate foot support for at least 10 minutes at a time twice each day at exactly the same times each day, so that a bowel rhythm could be established. A kitchen timer was suggested as a monitoring device. They were allowed to stay longer than 10 minutes if they wished, and were told they could read or listen to the radio, and that they could use the bathroom additionally at other times of the day. The two scheduled visits were to become a habitual routine and were not dependent upon whether or not the child needed to use the bathroom or had previous bowel movements. Children under eight were reinforced for toilet utilization through the use of a wall chart upon which they were given a star for each sitting. A contract was arranged whereby a certain number of stars would earn a prize.

Close monitoring and support was offered the family. A physician was available each morning by telephone to give advice. The children were seen three weeks after the initial clean-out. Further contacts were scheduled every four to eight weeks, depending upon the degree of persistence of the disorder. During these follow-up visits there were discussions of the child's muscle control and training program, as well as a physical examination. The child was also encouraged to talk about other issues in his or her life, and to review some of the past problems and strategies that occurred with respect to the encopresis. For those few cases where the physician felt the child was having difficulty dealing with feelings or coping with life stresses, psychological or psychiatric assistance was obtained.

At the end of one year, outcome data were available for 110 of the 127 children. Of these, 51 percent had not had "accidents" for more than six months. Another 27 percent showed marked improvement and were having only rare episodes of soiling. Fourteen percent of the children showed some improvement, but continued to have incontinence, while 8 percent showed no improvement whatsoever during the treatment year. The duration of encopresis at the onset of treatment (mean duration of three years), was not found to be significantly related to the success of treatment. Treatment failure was associated with children who had frequent "accidents" in school or at night, had very severe constipation and incontinence, showed reading or learning problems, and/or who showed signs of fearlessness, excessive moodiness, and disobedience. It was also found that the willingness of the parents and child to conform to the counseling program was a major determinant of successful or unsuccessful outcome in this study. The authors conclude that children who exhibit multiple problems other than encopresis, that is, learning, behavioral, and developmental difficulties, might need a broader interdisciplinary management approach.

Mercer (1967) studied 138 children for whom constipation was the primary problem that led to consultation at a medical center.

Excluded from the study were children with Hirschsprung's disease, cerebral palsy, and mental retardation. Analysis of the data revealed that 4 percent of the children had problems of acute constipation (disorder was of short duration and it responded quickly to simple enemas), 14 percent were found to have a disease causing the constipation (such as severe anal fissures), 17 percent had simple constipation, and 65 percent had psychogenic constipation. Children were considered to have simple constipation when there was no soiling, no evidence of severe emotional disturbance on the part of the child, and when the constipation subsided easily with simple measures of treatment. Most of these children were two or three years of age, and had a history of hard, dry stools which seemed related to the introduction of regular milk in the diet. The children with hard, dry stools responded well to the introduction of stool softeners (which are of little value with cases of psychogenic constipation).

Soiling was characteristic of 55 percent of the psychogenic cases. *Soiling* is defined by Mercer as the constant involuntary seepage of feces, and is differentiated from *encopresis* which he defines as the voluntary or involuntary passage of an ordinary bowel movement into the clothing. The latter was comparatively rare in this study, accounting for only four of the cases. When soiling occurs one can always assume the presence of a huge mass of feces in the rectum and the sigmoid colon. When this mass is removed, the soiling will always cease until such time as there has been a reaccumulation of the feces. Soiling does not occur in Hirschsprung's disorder despite the accumulation of massive amounts of feces.

Emotional disturbance was prominent among these children, their parents, or both. The children were characteristically tense, insecure, and anxious. Some were hostile, defiant, and controlling. Many of the children were lonely persons. The author notes, however, that often these signs of emotional disturbance disappear when the constipation is relieved. It seems that, for some cases, the constipation is the cause of the emotional disturbance and not the effect. Early toilet training (before 18 months) was found to be an etiologic factor in only 17 percent of the cases, and coercive training seemed present in only seven cases. Nineteen mothers were noted to be obviously neurotic and obsessed with the child's feces. In a few cases the constipation seemed related to stressful life events, such as the mother's remarriage, the birth of a sibling, or the first attendence at school.

Withholding of feces was a main feature at times. These children were often observed to cross their legs, stand rigidly upright, get red in the face and hold firmly to the furniture while waiting for the peristaltic sensation to pass away. This was often misinterpreted as an effort to produce a bowel movement. Another typical habit was the act of depositing feces in odd places around the house and out in the yard. Thirty-four of the children had a significant history of pain on defecation, with the passage of blood, which suggested the presence of an anal fissure at one time. For many of the children, a progression was noted from simple constipation in infancy with hard, dry stools, through a normal period of resistance to toilet training, to a severe problem of withholding, impaction, and soiling.

Although physicians have not been particularly successful in treating psychogenic constipation, the author recommends the following steps. First the fecal impaction must be removed by enemas. The Fleet enema is the most effective and easiest to use. Two consecutive adult-size enemas should be given each night and each morning until the bowel is empty. In some cases it is helpful to instill 3 or 4 ounces of mineral oil into the rectum to be retained overnight, followed by two enemas in the morning. Digital breaking and removal of an impaction is rarely necessary. Once the bowel is cleansed, mineral oil is a great therapeutic aid. Ordinary mineral oil covered with an ounce or two of orange juice is quite affective. The key to the use of mineral oil is that it must be used in large quantities, such as starting with 15 ml. five times daily and increasing the dose if necessary. It is important to get enough mineral oil into the child so that he actually complains that the oil is leaking out of the anus. The dosage is then reduced just enough to stop this leakage. The author feels that there is no danger of a vitamin deficiency if the bowel is saturated with oil for a limited period of time.

The third and most important aspect of treatment is to attempt to establish a routine bowel habit. Some effective techniques for toilet training are discussed in Chapter 3.

5

Summary and Conclusions

Encopresis is an extremely disturbing childhood disorder, the impact of which can be profound and long-lasting. Traditionally it has been the "great untalked-about topic" for parents and child-care professionals alike. The disorder seems to have a multiple etiology, and to be the culmination of a complex interaction between physiological predispositions (as evidenced by constipation in infancy), life events, parental childrearing practices, and other psychosocial and developmental factors. Regardless of the causative elements, the incidence of encopresis is roughly the same throughout the world, that is, 1.5 percent of the child population. Most often encopresis is psychogenic in nature and characterized by retention of feces which leads to chronic constipation.

The resistance of encopresis to many forms of management has been well recognized. Recently, however, there has been a pronounced upsurge of interest in this disorder by child therapists. A high success rate in treating this dysfunction has resulted from recent advances in treatment methods. Perhaps the primary conclusion that is apparent from the diverse approaches that have proven successful is the need for the clinician to be pluralistic in conceptual bases and in resulting observational methods and intervention techniques.

TECHNICAL ECLECTICISM

The individual child operates under a complex system of modalities–cognitive, imagery, physiological, social, and emotional–that must be integrated for optimal functioning. The need for the clinician to be flexible—to have the ability to move from one modality to another, and to combine modalities for effective treatment, is becoming increasingly obvious. This means that the child therapist must be familiar with diverse conceptual frameworks, and be skilled in a variety of techniques. For some, this type of flexibility means giving up the rigid application of a constricted set of methods to every encopretic child. A model of such a comprehensive approach is the multimodal therapy of Lazarus (1976). He uses a variety of intervention modalities and techniques, and combines them in accord with the needs of an individual case. Lazarus maintains that therapists need to be skilled in at least seven intervention modalities: behavior, affect, sensation-school, imagery, cognition, interpersonal relationship, and drug-diet. Thus, he presents a rationale for the systematic application of "technical eclectism."

In a similar vein, Harrison (1978) maintains that child psychiatrists must be pluralistic in therapeutic orientations and not display an unvarying devotion to a particular technique with all patients. The goal of therapy is specificity and therapeutic differentiation, and this can only be achieved when one can bring to bear multifaceted modes of therapeutic intervention. Careful history taking and diagnostic assessment will help one decide which techniques should be combined for the particular case. For example, the GAP report (1973) outlines five cases of school refusal. In each instance, diagnostic assessment led directly to a rational selection of five different therapeutic methods, each designed to change a different aspect of the individual child's functioning. Harrison concludes that a comparable pluralistic, eclectic orientation is best for other childhood disorders such as encopresis.

In brief, then, *technical eclecticism* means being skilled in a variety of specific techniques, flexibly applying them to the individual case, and combining different techniques and/or modalities for optimal effectiveness.

ELEMENTS OF OPTIMAL TREATMENT

A review of the most successful studies conducted to date suggest that the following elements should be combined in treating the encopretic child:

1. Carefully assess the case and take a detailed history of the problem. Include a physical exam to rule out colonic impaction and any organic factors that may contribute to the soiling.

2. When colonic impaction is present it seems best to clean the child out early in treatment by the use of Dulcolax suppositories or Fleet enemas.

3. The trend is to use parents to administer the intervention, under supervision of an experienced therapist, in the home, so as to ensure generalization of results.

4. To overcome feelings of guilt, shame, and hopelessness, offer parents and child a plausible, nonblaming explanation of the causes of the disorder, within a supportive relationship with them. Show an empathic understanding of the child's plight and the parents' frustration.

5. Establish the expectation in the child and parents that due to their own efforts they will be successful within a realistic time period of about two to three months.

6. Knowledge of normal bowel function by all concerned is most helpful. So offer an understanding of the physiology of the bowel and, when appropriate, attribute the prime cause of the encopresis to weak colonic muscles.

7. Daily recording of accidents and appropriate eliminations, and posting these results, has been found to be essential for the success of behavioral methods.

8. An incentive program, that is, provision of rewards or pleasant consequences contingent upon bowel movements in the toilet and clean pants, has been found to be quite effective.

9. Counseling the parents as to effective toileting practices may be needed in some cases.

10. If the child is fearful of the toilet, the parents should be offered guidance as to how to desensitize the child to the toilet.

11. The child's cooperation and active involvement in the treatment should be solicited. The child can for example, be given the responsibility for recording on a display chart the daily successes and failures in regard to defecation. The child should also have some voice in deciding upon the choice of rewards for successes. Responsibility for cleaning self and clothing after soiling should also be the child's.

12. Training for the parents and child in administering enemas or suppositories in a nonadversive manner is often needed since this is frequently the cause of unsuccessful treatment.

13. Gradual fading out of incentives and/or cathartics and restoring them temporarily if symptoms reappear is a key to success.

14. Consistency by the parents in administering the program needs to be stressed, encouraged, and monitored by the therapist.

15. Often the child's underwear has to be numbered to prevent hiding attempts.

16. Encourage the child to follow a reasonable diet that is high in bulk or fiber content (fruit, vegetables, and bran) but be careful not to overdo this lest the opposite effect, diarrhea, occur. Bananas, rhubarb, figs, dates, and applesauce are also recommended. Junk food should be minimized and the child should be prompted to drink plenty of water.

17. An effort should be made to establish regular bowel habits, but not to the point of obsession or panic if the scheduled time is missed or the attempt is unsuccessful. Ample time should be allowed for defecation to occur, that is, about 10 to 15 minutes on the toilet.

18. Every effort should be made to help the child kick the laxative habit and regain control over his or her own bowels. There are some cases in which certain kinds of laxatives can be beneficial, but the drugs must be administered with care and close supervision by one who is skilled in their use. In most cases they will not be needed at all. Misuse can bring about diarrhea, motor paralysis, electrolyte imbalances, sodium intoxication, esophageal obstruction, and even prostration. Because of these hazards, Benson (1975) states that, "all measures designed to improve bowel habits and to naturally restore normal physiologic function should be employed before resorting to the ancillary use of drugs to help overcome constipation."

In summary, optimal treatment involves combining different techniques to meet the needs of the individual case, the minimum use of drugs—especially laxatives, minimum use of punishment and maximum use of rewards, regular and effective toilet habits, use of parents in the home environment, and the child's involvement in treatment.

FURTHER RESEARCH AND EXPERIMENTATION

Most of the available studies of constipation and encopresis are of the case study method. There is a pressing need for more valid experimental designs to evaluate treatment effectiveness, such as a random assignment of cases to experimental and control groups or to alternate treatment groups, reversal designs (ABAB), and the multiple baseline design. Typically, clinicians have simply reported the level of soiling prior to treatment and the level after intervention. These AB designs provide little evidence that observed changes are due to treatment rather than extraneous factors. There is also a need to study the possibility that differential treatment is needed for continuous vs. discontinous encopresis, and for longitudinal investigations of the natural history of encopresis and to look more carefully at the possibility of symptom substitution. Until such studies are conducted, any conclusions as to optimal treatment interventions, including those previously mentioned, must be regarded as tentative.

Glossary

aliment. Anything that nourishes; food.

alimentary canal. The passage in the body that food goes through: it extends from the mouth through the esophagus, stomach, and intestines to the anus.

anal fissures. Small cracks or lesions in the skin of the anus which are painful, especially when the child is having a bowel movement. The cause is usually constipation and the passage of large, hard stools.

anus. The opening at the lower end of the alimentary canal.

barium enema. A solution of barium sulfate is inserted through the rectum into the colon to aid in taking X-ray pictures of the large intestine. Such X-rays can help identify any anatomical or neurological deficits that may be present in the colon.

bolus. Portion of masticated food.

borborygmus. A gurgling, splashing sound heard over the large intestine; intestinal flatus.

bowel. An intestine.

bowel movement. The passing of waste matter from the large intestine.

cecum. Beginning of the large intestine, consisting of a pouch situated on the right side of the body, about 2 x 3 inches, adjoining the ascending colon. Attached to the cecum is the vermiform appendix, about 3–4 inches long, function unknown.

"call to stool". Food residue reaching the rectum causes a sensation referred to as the "call to stool" or the urge to defecate. This sensation is related to periodic increase in pressure within the rectum and contraction of its muscles.

cathartic. An active purgative, usually producing several bowel evacuations. Includes laxatives and enemas.

chyme. The mixture of partly digested food and digestive secretions found in the stomach and small intestine during digestion of a meal; it is a varicolored, thick, but nearly liquid mass.

Colace. A stool-softener composed of dioctyl sodium sulfosuccinate. By its surface-active properties, Colace keeps stools soft for easy, natural passage. Not a laxative, thus not habit forming. Does not irritate intestinal tract. Useful in constipation due to hard stools. The effect on stools after liquid Colace is usually not apparent until one to three days after the first dose.

colitis. A disorder in which the lining of part of the colon, or large intestine, is inflammed. There is usually a correlation between colitis and depression or anxiety. In the early stages, colitis is characterized by abdominal cramps or pain, diarrhea, and the need to eliminate several times a day.

colon. Part of the large intestine from the cecum to the rectum. The colon averages 4–6 feet in length. The first portion of *ascending colon* extends from the cecum to the under surface of the liver where it turns to the left as the *transverse colon.* Its bend is the right colic or hepatic flexure. The transverse colon passes horizontally to the left to the region of the spleen where it turns downward as the *descending colon.* This turn is the *splenic flexure.* The descending colon continues downward on the left side of the abdomen until it reaches the pelvic brim and curves like the letter S and is placed in front of the sacrum to become the *rectum.* This S-shaped section is known as the *"sigmoid colon."* The rectum, about 6–8 inches long, passes downward to terminate in the lower opening of the tract, the *anus* or *anal opening.*

continuous encopresis. Child has never developed bowel control for any sustained period.

constipation. A disorder causing decreased frequency of bowel movements, resulting in waste matter remaining in the colon and becoming dry and difficult to expel.

coprolagnia. An erotic satisfaction at the sight or odor of excreta.

coprolalia. A morbid desire to use obscene words in ordinary conversation.

coprolith. Hard fecal matter.

coprology. Examination of the feces.

coproma. Accumulation of feces in the rectum.

coprophagy. The eating of excrement.

coprophobia. A morbid disgust at the sight of filth of any kind.

dilate. To make wider or larger; cause to expand or swell.

discontinuous encopresis. Child initially developed control over defecation but subsequently became incontinent.

diverticulitis. Inflammation of the small sacs (diverticula), or out-pouchings, that may be found along the small or large intestine. Symptoms include pain in the lower abdomen accompanying bowel movements, abdominal bloating, and frequent urge to eliminate followed by constipation. Called "irritable bowel" because of alternating attacks of constipation and diarrhea.

Dulcolax. A contact laxative acting directly on the colonic mucosa to produce normal peristalsis throughout the large intestine. Its unique mode of action permits either oral or rectal administration. Because of its gentleness and reliability of action without side effects, Dulcolax may be used whenever constipation is a problem.

The drug, administered rectally is negligibly absorbed. Dulcolax has been extremely effective in the management of chronic constipation. By gradually lengthening the interval between doses as colonic tone improves, the drug has been found to be effective in redeveloping proper bowel hygiene.

duodenum. The first section of the small intestine, between the stomach and the jejunum.

dyschezia. Constipation due to habitual neglect to respond to stimulus to defecate. The rectum tends to be constantly full of feces, small amounts of which are expelled at short intervals without ever producing complete evacuation.

dyspepsia. Pain, or any uncomfortable symptom associated with the function of digestion.

encopresis. Involuntary discharge of feces in a child four years or older.

enema. Injection of water, either plain or containing various drugs, into the rectum and colon to empty the lower intestine.

enuresis. Involuntary discharge of urine (after four years of age).

epithelium. The layer of cells forming the epidermis of the skin and the surface layer of mucous and serous membranes.

fecaloma. A large mass of accumulated feces in the rectum resembling a tumor.

feces. Stools; excreta; dejecta; excrement. Body waste, such as food residue, bacteria, epithelium, and mucus, discharged from the bowels by way of the anus.

flatus. Gas in digestive tract.

gastrocolonic reflex. Increase in colonic motor activity following a meal or intake of fluid.

gastroileal reflex. Physiologic relaxation of ileocecal valve resulting from food in stomach.

gastrointestinal. Pertaining to stomach and intestine.

GI tract. Gastrointestinal system.

hemorrhoids. Ruptured or distended veins located around the anus.

iatrogenic disorder. Condition involving adverse effects induced by a physician in the case of patients. For example, injudicious, prolonged use of laxatives and suppositories can result in chronic constipation in a child.

ileocecal valve. Sphincter muscles which guard the aperture of the ileum at the cecum, where the small intestines open into the ascending colon. It prevents food material from reentering the small intestines.

ileum. The lowest part of the small intestine, opening into the large intestine.

incontinence. Inability to control urination and/or defecation.

inspissated. Thickened by absorption, evaporation or dehydration of fluid.

intestines. The lower part of the alimentary canal, extending from the stomach to the anus and consisting of a convoluted upper part (small intestine) and a lower part of greater diameter (large intestine).

jejunum. The middle part of the small intestine, between the duodenum and the ileum.

lactase. An intestinal enzyme needed to digest lactose, the sugar found in milk.

laxative. A mildly purgative medicine which produces one or two bowel movements without pain.

masticate. To chew food with the teeth to prepare for swallowing.

megacolon. Disorder of large intestine in which the colon becomes extremely dilated because of the presence of a large quantity of retained feces. Sometimes the entire abdominal cavity is filled. Seepage may occur because the child is so constipated that only liquid stools can bypass the blockage caused by hard impacted stools. When stools are finally passed (maybe once in several weeks) they often have an extremely foul odor. Rapid weight loss from lack of appetite is present in some cases.

Metamucil. Promotes natural elimination by adding bland, nonirritating bulk to the diet. It consists of a highly refined vegetable mucilloid of the psyllium seed. An equal amount of dextrose is added as a dispensing agent. Contraindications are intestinal obstruction, and fecal impaction.

neurogenic. Originating from disorder of the nerve cells or nervous impulses.

obstipation. Inability to move the bowels as a result of an obstructing lesion.

parineum. Part of the body between the scrotum and anus in the male. It consists mainly of skin and muscle.

peristalsis. The rhythmic, wavelike motion of the walls of the alimentary canal, consisting of alternate muscular contractions and dilations that move the contents of the tube onward into the rectum where the waste is stored. This signals the sphincter muscle of anus to relax and open.

proctologist. One who specializes in diseases of the rectum and anus.

proctosigmoidoscopy. Direct visual examination of the rectum and the sigmoid colon, performed with the aid of a hollow metal tube called a *proctoscope.* A light on one end of the tube permits the inner lining of the bowel walls to be seen directly.

psychogenic. Originating mainly from psychological factors.

purgative. An agent that will cause watery evacuation of the intestinal contents. Examples: castor oil, calomel, cascara sagrada, enemas.

rectum. The lowest end of the large intestine, extending from the sigmoid flexure to the anus.

rewards. One can strengthen and accelerate desired behavior by using rewards or "positive reinforcers." Positive reinforcers of biological significance are food, water, and physical contact. Positive reinforcers of *acquired* significance are praise, grades, money, etc.

scatology. Scientific study and analysis of the feces.

scatoma. Mass of inspissated feces in colon or rectum resembling an abdominal tumor.

scybalum (pl. : scybala). A hard, rounded mass of fecal matter.

segmentation. Division of the intestine and the chyme within it into segments by contraction of circular muscle fibers.

Senokot Suppositories. A prompt-acting, rectal-route laxative that may be used in place of an enema. These suppositories combine gentle action with predictable results, usually inducing comfortable evacuation within 30 minutes to 2 hours (without reported irritation or "explosive" elimination of feces).

Senokot Tablets. A natural laxative and stool softener combination, these tablets consist of standardized senna concentrate (laxative) and diotyl sodium sulfosuccinate (stool softener). Best administered at bedtime, the tablets take 8–10 hours to produce results.

sigmoid flexure. The last curving part of the colon, ending in the rectum. S-shaped.

spastic. Resembling, or of the nature of spasms or convulsions.

sphincter. A ring-shaped muscle that surrounds the natural opening of the anus and can open or close it by expanding or contracting.

stenosis. Constriction or narrowing of a passage or orifice.

supine. Lying on the back, or with the face upward.

suppository (glycerine). A semisolid substance for insertion into the rectum to assist evacuation. Shaped like a cylinder it contains about 70 percent glycerine, which has lubricating and stool softening properties.

References

Abrahams, D. Treatment of encopresis with Imipramine. *American Journal of Psychiatry,* 1963, **119**, 891–892.

Achenbach, T.M. and Lewis, M. A proposed model for clinical research and its application to encopresis and enuresis. *Journal of Child Psychiatry,* 1971, **10**, 535–554.

Andolfi, M. A structural approach to a family with an encopretic child. *Journal of Marriage and Family Counseling,* 1978, **4**, 25–29.

Anthony, E.J. An experimental approach to the psychopathology of childhood. *British Journal of Medical Psychology*, 1957, **30**, 146–175.

Ashkenazi, Z. The treatment of encopresis using a discriminative stimulus and positive reinforcement. *Journal of Behavior Therapy and Experimental Psychiatry*, 1975, **6**, 155–157.

Ayllon, T., Simon, S.J., and Wildman, R.W. Instructions and reinforcement in the elimination of encopresis: A case study. *Journal of Behavior Therapy and Experimental Psychiatry,* 1975, **6**, 235–238.

Azrin, N.H. and Foxx, R.M. A rapid method of toilet training the institutionalized retarded. *Journal of Applied Behavior Analysis,* 1971, **4**, 89–99.

Azrin, N.H. and Foxx, R.M. *Toilet training in less than a day.* New York, Simon and Schuster, 1974.

Bach, R. and Moylan, J.J. Parents administer behavior therapy for inappropriate urination and encopresis: A case study. *Journal of Behavior Therapy and Experimental Psychiatry,* 1975, **6**, 239–241.

Baird, M. Characteristic interaction patterns in families of encopretic children. *Bulletin of the Menninger Clinic,* 1974, **38**, 144–153.

Bakwin, H. Constipation in children. *Pediatric Clinics of North America,* 1956, **3**, 127–136.

Balson, P.M. Case Study: Encopresis: A case with symptom substitution. *Behavior Therapy,* 1973, **4**, 134–136.

Barrett, B.H. Behavior modification in the home: Parents adapt laboratory-developed tactics to bowel-train a 5 ½-year-old. *Psychotherapy: Theory, Research and Practice,* 1969, **6**, 172–176.

Bell, A.I., and Levine, M.I. The psychologic aspects of pediatric practice: Causes and treatment of chronic constipation. *Pediatrics,* 1954, **14**, 259.

Bellman, M. Studies in encopresis. *Acta Pediatrica Scandinavia,* 1966, **170**, (Supp.)

Bemporad, J.R., Pfeifer, C.M., Gibbs, L., Cortner, R.H., and Bloom, W. Characteristics of encopretic patients and their families. *Journal of Child Psychiatry,* 1971, **10**, 272–292.

Benjamin, L. Serdahely, W., and Geppert, T. Night training through parents implicit use of operant conditioning. *Child Development,* 1971, **42**, 963–966.

Benson, J.A. Simple chronic constipation: Pathophysiology and management. *Postgraduate Medicine,* 1975, **57**, 55.

Berg, L. and Jones, K.V. Functional fecal incontinence in children. *Archives of Diseases of Childhood,* 1964, **39**, 465–472.

Blatz, W.E. and Bott, H. *Parents and the pre-school child.* New York, William Morrow, 1929.

Blechman, E.A. Home-based treatment of encopresis: Pleasant, and successful. Paper presented at the 49th annual meeting of the Eastern Psychological Association, March, 1978.

Bodian, M. Chronic constipation in children with particular reference to Hirschsprung's disease. *Practitioner,* 1952, **169**, 517–529.

Boucharlat, J., Salomon, R., Pellat, J., and Wolf, R. L'Encopresie (abstract). *Excerpta Medica: Psychiatry,* 1970, **23**, 574–575.

Brazelton, T.B. A child oriented approach to toilet training. *Pediatrics,* 1962, **29**, 121.

Browne, D. Contributions to a discussion on megacolon and megarectum. *Proceedings of the Royal Society of Medicine,* 1961, **54**, 1055–1056.

Burns, C. Encopresis in children. *British Medical Journal,* 1941, **2**, 767–769.

Butler, J.F. Treatment of encopresis by overcorrection. *Psychological Reports,* 1977, **40**, 639–646.

Caldwell, B.M. The effects of infant care. In Hoffman, L.W. and Hoffman, M.L. (Eds.), *Review of Child Development Research.* Vol. **I**, New York, Russell Sage, 1964.

Call, J.D., Christianson, M., Penrose, F.R., and Backlar, M. Psychogenic megacolon in three pre-school boys: A study of etiology through collaborative treatment of child and parents. *American Journal of Orthopsychiatry,* 1963, **33**, 923–928.

Cashmore, G.R. The reduction of soiling behavior in an 11-year-old boy with the parent as therapist. *New Zealand Medical Journal,* 1976, **84**, 238–239.

Chapman, A.H., and Loeb, D.G. Psychosomatic gastrointestinal problems. *A.M.A. Journal of Diseases of Children,* 1955, **12**, 717–724.

Coekin, M., and Gairdner, D. Fecal incontinence in children. *British Medical Journal,* 1960, **2**, 1175.

Cohen, T.B. Observations on school children in the People's Republic of China. *Journal of Child Psychiatry,* 1977, **16**, 165–173.

Cone, T.E. Jr. How Henoch treated children with encopresis. *Pediatrics,* 1970, **46**, 802.

Conger, J.C. The treatment of encopresis by the management of social consequences. *Behavior Therapy,* 1970, **1**, 386–390.

Davenport, H.W. *Physiology of the digestive tract.* Chicago, Year Book Medical Publishers, 1971.

Davidson, M. Constipation and fecal incontinence. *Pediatric Clinics of North America,* 1958, **5**, 749–757.

Davidson, M. and Bauer, C.H. Studies of distal colonic motility in children. *Pediatrics,* 1959, **21**, 746–761.

Davidson, M., Kugle, M.M., and Bauer, C.H. Diagnosis and management in children with severe and protracted constipation and obstipation. *Journal of Pediatrics,* 1963, **62**, 261–275.

Davis, H.M. *et al.* A behavioral programme for the modification of encopresis. *Child Care Health Development,* 1976, **2**, 273–282.

Davis, H.M. *et al.* A pilot study of encopretic children treated by behavior modification. *Practitioner,* 1977, **219**, 228–230.

Dayan, M. Toilet training retarded children in a state residential institution. *Mental Retardation,* 1964, **2**, 116–117.

Derezin, M. Laxatives and fecal modifiers. *American Family Physician,* 1974, **10**, 126.

de Vries, M.W., and de Vries, M.R. Cultural relativity of toilet training readiness. A perspective from East Africa. *Pediatrics,* 1977, **60**, 170–177.

Doleys, D.M., and Arnold, S. Treatment of childhood encopresis by full cleanliness training. *Mental Retardation,* 1975, **13**, 14–16.

Duhamel, J., Bensaid, F., and Koupernick, C. Apropos de 33 cas d'encopresie. *Archives Francoise Pediatrica,* 1957, **14**, 1031–1049.

Easson, W.M. Encropesis—psychogenic soiling. *Canadian Medical Association Journal,* 1960, **82**, 624–628.

Edelman, R.I. Operant conditioning treatment of encopresis. *Journal of Behavior Therapy and Experimental Psychiatry,* 1971, **2**, 71–73.

Eller, H. Uber die Encopresis im Kindersalter. *Mschr. Kinderheilk,* 1960, **108**, 415–421.

Ellis, N.R. Toilet training the severely defective patient, an S-R reinforcement analysis. *American Journal of Mental Deficiency,* 1963, **68**, 98–103.

Engel, B.T. *et al.* Operant conditioning of rectosphincteric responses in the treatment of fecal incontinence. *The New England Journal of Medicine,* 1974, **290**, 646–649.

Epstein, L.H. and McCoy, J.F. Bladder and bowel control in Hirschsprung's Disease. *Journal of Behavior Therapy and Experimental Psychiatry,* 1977, **8**, 97–99.

Ferinden, W., and Van Handel, D. Elimination of soiling behavior in an elementary school child through the application of aversive techniques. *Journal of School Psychology,* 1970, **8**, 267–269.

Fowler, G.B. Incontinence of feces in children. *American Journal of Obstetrics and Disorders of Women and Children,* 1882, **15**, 984–988.

Foxx, R.M. and Azrin, N.H. Dry pants: A rapid method of toilet training children. *Behavior Research and Therapy,* 1973 a, **11**, 435–442.

Foxx, R.M. and Azrin, N.H. *Toilet training the retarded.* Champaign, Ill., Research Press, 1973 b.

Fraiberg, S.H. *The magic years.* New York, Charles Scribner's Sons, 1959.

Freeman, B.J., and Pribble, W. Elimination of inappropriate toileting behavior by overcorrection. *Psychological Reports,* 1974, **35**, 802.

Freud, A. *Normality and pathology in childhood: Assessments of development.* New York, International Universities Press, 1965.

Fries, M.E. and Woolf, P.J. Some hypotheses on the role of the congenital activity type in personality development. *The Psychoanalytic Study of the Child,* 1953, **8**, 48–62.

Frommer, E.A. Depressive illness in childhood. In *Recent developments in affective disorders,* A. Copper and A. Walk (Eds.). *British Journal of Psychiatry,* Special Publication No. **2**, 117–136.

Gairdner, D. Incontinence of urine or feces. *British Medical Journal,* 1965, **54**, 91–94.

Garrard, S.D. and Richmond, J.B. Psychogenic megacolon manifested by fecal soiling. *Pediatrics,* 1952, **10**, 474–481.

Gavanski, M. Treatment of non-retentive secondary encopresis with Imipramine and psychotherapy. *Canadian Medical Association Journal,* 1971, **104**, 46–48.

Gelber, H. and Meyer, V. Behavior therapy and encopresis. *Behavior Research and Therapy,* 1965, **2**, 227–231.

Giles, D.K. and Montrose, M.W. Toilet training institutionalized severe retardates: An application of operant behavior modification techniques. *American Journal of Mental Deficiency,* 1960, **78**, 766–780.

Gott, H. Incontinentia alvi und Enkopresis im Kindersalter. *Deutsch Med. Wschr.,* 1959, **84**, 112–115.

Grinker, R.R. Hypothalamic functions in psychosomatic interrelations. *Psychosomatic Medicine,* 1939, **1**, 19–47.

Grosick, J.P. Effects of operant conditioning in modification of incontinence in neuropsychiatric geriatric patients. *Nursing Research,* 1968, **17**, 304–311.

Group for the Advancement of Psychiatry. *From diagnosis to treatment.* New York, GAP Report 87, **8**, 520–661, 1973.

Hall, M.B. Encopresis in children. *British Medical Journal,* 1941, **2**, 890.

Hallgren, B. Enuresis. *Acta Psychiatrica Neurology Scandinavia Supplement,* 1957, **32** (114), 1–159.

Halpern, W.I. The child guidance clinic in a community mental health center. *Community Mental Health Journal,* 1974, **10**, 292–300.

Halpern, W.I. The treatment of encopretic children. *Journal of Child Psychiatry,* 1977, **16**, 478–499.

Halpern, W.I. and Kissel, S. *Human resources for troubled children.* New York, Wiley-Interscience, 1976.

Harrison, S.I. Child psychiatry perspectives: Therapeutic choice in child psychiatry. *Journal of Child Psychiatry,* 1978, **17**, 165–172.

Hein, H.A., and Beerends, J.J. Who should accept primary responsibility for the encopretic child? *Clinical Pediatrics,* 1978, **17**, 67–70.

Henoch, E. *Lectures on children's diseases: A handbook for practitioners and students.* (Translated from the Fourth German edition by John Thomson). London, New Sydenhem, Vol. **II**, 180–181, 1889.

Hilburn, W.B. Encopresis in childhood. *Journal Kentucky Medical Association,* 1968, **66**, 978–982.

Hindley, C.B., Fillozat, A.M., Klackenberg, G., Nicolet-Meister, D., and Sand, E.A. Some differences in infant feeding and elimination training in five European longitudinal samples. *Journal of Child Psychology and Psychiatry,* 1965, **6**, 179–201.

Hoag, J.M., Norriss, N.G., Himeno, E.T. and Jacobs, J. The encopretic child and his family. *Journal of Child Psychiatry,* 1971, **10**, 242–256.

Horne, A.M. Teaching parents a reinforcement program. *Elementary School Guidance and Counseling Journal,* 1974, **9**, 102–107.

Houle, T.A. The use of positive reinforcement and aversive conditioning in the treatment of encopresis: A case study. *Devereux Forum,* 1974, **9**, 7–14.

Hundziak, M., Maurer, R.A., and Watson, L.S. Operant conditioning in toilet training of severely mentally retarded boys. *Americal Journal of Mental Deficiency,* 1965, **70**, 120–124.

Huschka, M. The child's response to coercive bowel training. *Psychosomatic Medicine,* 1942, **4**, 301–308.

Ilg, F.L., and Ames, L.B. *Child Behavior.* New York, Harper and Row, 1955.

Jekelius, E. Incontinenta alvi im kindersalter. *Arch. Kinderheilk,* 1936, **109**, 129–130.

Johnson, J.H., and Bourgondien, M.E. Behavior therapy and encopresis: A selective review of the literature. *Journal of Clinical Child Psychology,* 1977, Spring, 15–19.

Jost, H., and Sontag, L.W. The genetic factor in autonomic nervous system function. *Psychosomatic Medicine,* 1944, **6**, 308–310.

Kanner, L. *Child Psychiatry* (2nd Ed.) Springfield, Ill., Thomas, 1953.

Katz, J. Enuresis and encopresis. *Medical Journal of Australia,* 1972, **1**, 127–130.

Keat, D.B. Multimodal counseling with children: Treating the basic id. *Pennsylvania Personnel and Guidance Association Journal,* 1976, **4**, 21–25.

Keehn, J.D. Brief case report: Reinforcement therapy of incontinence. *Behavior Research and Therapy,* 1965, **2**, 239.

Kellerman, J. Childhood encopresis: A multimodal therapeutic approach. *Psychiatric Opinion,* 1977, **14**, 39–43.

Kohlenberg, R.J. Operant conditioning of human anal sphincter pressure. *Journal of Applied Behavior Analysis,* 1973, **6**, 201–208.

Kottmeier, P.K. and Clatworthy, H.W. Aganglionic and functional megacolon in children—a diagnostic dilemma. *Pediatrics,* 1965, **36**, 572.

Krug, O. and Stuart, B.L. Collaborative treatment of mother and boy with fecal retention, soiling, and a school phobia. *Case Studies in Childhood Emotional Disabilities.* Vol **II**, New York, American Orthopsychiatric Assoc., 1956.

Lal, H. and Lindsley, O.R. Therapy of chronic constipation in a young child by rearranging social contingencies. *Behavior Research and Therapy,* 1968, **6**, 484–485.

Lambley, P. Treatment of a severe case of encopresis by a system-based operant method. *Psychotherapy: Theory, Research and Practice,* 1976, **13**, 286–289.

Lazarus, A.A. (Ed.) *Multimodal Behavior Therapy.* New York, Springer, 1976.

Lee, C.M. and Bebb, K.C. Pathogenesis and clinical management of megacolon, with emphasis on the fallacy of the term "idiopathic." *Surgery,* 1951, **30,** 1026–1048.

Lehman, E. Psychogenic incontinence of feces (encopresis) in children. *American Journal of Diseases of Childhood,* 1944, **68**, 190–199.

Le Vine, B. and Le Vine, R. Nyansongo: A Gusii community in Kenya. In B. Whiting (ed.), *Six cultures: Studies of child rearing.* New York, Wiley, 1963.

Levine, M.D. Children with encopresis: A descriptive analysis. *Pediatrics,* 1975, **56,** 412.

Levine, M.D. and Bakow, H. Children with encopresis: A study of treatment outcome. *Pediatrics,* 1976, **58,** 845–852.

Lieberman, A.D. Confirmation of Henoch's treatment of encopresis. *Pediatrics,* 1971, **48,** 674–675.

Lifshitz, M. and Chovers, A. Encopresis among Israeli kibbutz children. *Israeli Annals of Psychiatry,* 1972, **10**, 326–340.

Logan, D.L. and Garner, D. Effective behavior modification for reducing chronic soiling. *American Journal for the Deaf,* 1971, **116**, 382–384.

MacNamara, M. Notes on a case of lifelong encopresis. *British Journal of Medical Psychology,* 1965, **38**, 333–338.

Madsen, C.H., Hoffman, M., Thomas, D.R., Karapsak, E., and Madsen, C.K. Comparison of toilet training techniques in social learning in childhood. In D.M. Gelfand (ed.), *Readings in theory and application,* pp. 124–132. Belmont, California, Brooks Cole, 1969.

Madsen, C.R. Positive reinforcement in the toilet training of a normal child: A case report. In L. Krasner, and L.P. Ullman (eds.), *Case studies in behavior modification,* pp. 305–307, New York; Holt, Rinehart and Winston, 1965.

McDonagh, M.J. Is operant conditioning effective in reducing enuresis and encopresis in children? *Perspectives on Psychiatric Care,* 1971, **9**, 17–23.

McGregor, M. Chronic constipation in children. In R. McKeith and J. Sandler (eds.), *Psychosomatic aspects of pediatrics,* Oxford, England, Pergamon Press, 1961.

McTaggart, A. and Scott, M. A review of twelve cases of encopresis. *Journal of Pediatrics,* 1959, **54**, 762–768.

Mercer, R.D. Constipation. *Pediatric Clinics of North America,* 1967, **14**, 175–188.

Mercer, R.D. and Turnbull, R.B. The diagnosis of constipation in infants and children. *Diseases of Colon and Rectum,* 1961, **4**, 33.

Mittlemann, B. Motility in infants, children and adults. *The Psychoanalytic Study of the Child,* 1954, **9**, 142–177.

Musicco, N. Encopresis: A good result in a boy with UTP (uridine-5-triphosphate). *American Journal of Proctology,* 1977, **28**, 43–46.

Neale, D.H. Behavior therapy and encopresis in children. *Behavior Research and Therapy,* 1963, **1**, 139–149.
Niedermeyer, K. and Parnitzke, K.H. Die enkopresis. *Z. Kinderheilk,* 1963, **87**, 404–431.
Nussey, A.M. Encopresis in children. *British Medical Journal,* 1941, **2**, 927.
Olatawura, M.O. Encopresis: A review of thirty-two cases. *Acta Paediatrica Scandinavia,* 1973, **62**, 358–364.
Oxenius, K. Uber Enkopresis. *Kinderärtzth Praxis,* 1949, **17**, 384.
Perdini, B.C. and Perdini, D.T. Reinforcement procedures in the control of encopresis. *Psychological Reports,* 1971, **28**, 937–938.
Perzan, R.S., Boulander, F., and Fischer, D.G. Complex factors in inhibition of defecation: A review and case study. *Journal of Behavior Therapy and Experimental Psychiatry,* 1972, **3**, 129–133.
Peterson, D.R. and London, P. Neobehavioristic psychotherapy: Quasi-hypnotic suggestion and multiple reinforcement in the treatment of a case of postinfantile dyscopresis. *Psychological Record,* 1964, **14**, 469–474.
Peterson, D.R. and London, P. A role for cognition in the behavioral treatment of a child's eliminative disturbance. In L. Krasner and L.P. Ullmann (eds.), *Case Studies in Behavior Modification,* 289–296, New York, Holt, Rinehart and Winston, 1965.
Pinkerton, P. Psychogenic megacolon in children: The implications of bowel negativism. *Archives Diseases of Childhood,* 1958, **33**, 371–380.
Plachetta, K.E. Encopresis: A case study utilizing contracting, scheduling and self-charting. *Journal of Behavior Therapy and Experimental Psychiatry,* 1976, **7**, 195–196.
Pototsky, C. Die Enkopresis. In: *Psychogenese und psycotherapie körperlicher symptome,* O. Schwarz (ed.), Berlin, Springer, 1925.
Priesel, R. and Siegel, J. Chronische obstipation als ursache für incontinentia alvi. *Arch. Kinderheilk,* 1936, **107**, 133–136.
Prugh, D.G. Child experience and colonic disorders. *Annals New York Academy of Science,* 1954, **58**, 355–376.
Quarti, C. and Renaud, J. A new treatment of constipation by conditioning: A preliminary report. In C.M. Franks (ed.), *Conditioning Techniques in Clinical Practice and Research.* New York, Springer, 1964.
Ravitch, M.M. Pseudo Hirschsprung's disease. *Annals of Surgery,* 1958, **147**, 781–795.
Richard, H.C. and Griffin, J.L. Reducing soiling behavior in a therapeutic summer camp. In J.D. Krumboltz and C.E. Thoresen (eds.), *Behavioral Counseling Cases and Techniques.* New York, Holt, Rinehart and Winston, 1969.
Richmond, J.B. in *Psychosomatic aspects of gastrointestinal illness in childhood.* Report of the Forty-Fourth Ross Conference on Pediatric Research, Columbus, Ross Labs, 1963, p. 85.
Richmond, J.B., Eddy, E.J. and Garrard, S.D. The syndrome of fecal soiling and megacolon. *American Journal of Orthopsychiatry,* 1954, **24**, 391–401.
Ross, E.A. A toilet training difficulty. *Psychoanalysis,* 1953, **2**, 75–76.

Sachs, L.J. An unusual object choice during the oedipal phase. *Psychoanalytic Quarterly,* 1974, **43**, 477–492.

Schaefer, C.E. Treating psychogenic encopresis: A case study. *Psychological Reports,* 1978, **42**, 98.

Scott, E.A. Treatment of encopresis in a classroom setting: A case study. *British Journal of Educational Psychology,* 1977, **47**, 199–202.

Sears, R.R., Maccoby, E.E., and Levin, H. *Patterns of child-rearing.* New York, Harper and Row, 1957.

Segall, A. Report of a constipated child with fecal withholding. *American Journal of Orthopsychiatry,* 1957, **27**, 820–826.

Seymour, F.W. The treatment of encopresis using behavior modification. *Australian Pediatric Journal,* 1976, **12**, 326–329.

Shane, M. Encopresis in a latency boy. *The Psychoanalytic Study of the Child,* 1967, **22**, 296–314.

Sheinbein, M. A triadic-behavioral approach to encopresis. *Journal of Family Counseling,* 1975, **12**, 58–61.

Shirley, H.F. Encopresis in children. *Journal of Pediatrics,* 1938, **12**, 367–380.

Selander, P. and Torald, A. Enkopres. *Nordic Medicine,* 1964, **72**, 1110.

Silber, D.L. Encopresis: Discussion of etiology and management. *Clinical Pediatrics,* 1969, **8**, 225–231.

Silber, S. Encopresis: Rectal rebellion and anal anarchy? *American Society for Psychosomatic and Dental Medicine,* 1968, **15**, 97–106.

Stein, Z. and Susser, M. Social factors in the development of sphincter control. *Developmental Medicine and Child Neurology,* 1967, **9**, 692–706.

Stengel, A. Diseases of the intestines. In *Modern Medicine,* W. Osler (ed.), Philadelphia, Lea and Febiger, 1908, **5**, 363.

Sterba, E. Analysis of psychogenic constipation in a two-year old child. *The Psychoanalytic Study of the Child,* 1949, **3-4**, New York, International Universities Press.

Sullivan, D.B., Dickinson, D.D., and Wilson, J.L. The conservative management of fecal incontinence in children. *Journal of American Medical Association,* 1963, **185**, 664–666.

Swenson, O. Congenital megacolon (Hirschsprung's disease). *Pediatrics,* 1951, **8**, 542–547.

Szasz, T.S. Physiologic and psychodynamic mechanisms in constipation and diarrhea. *Psychosomatic Medicine,* 1951, **13**, 113–116.

Taichert, L.C. Childhood encopresis: A neuro-developmental family approach to management. *California Medical Journal,* 1971, **115**, 11.

Thiroloix, J. *Constipation: Its causes and cures.* New York, St. Martin's Press, 1976.

Thomas, A., Chess, S. and Birch, H.G. *Temperament and behavior disorders in Children.* New York, New York University Press, 1968.

Tomlinson, J.R. The treatment of bowel retention by operant procedures. *Journal of Behavior Therapy and Experimental Psychiatry.* 1970, **1**, 83–85.

Wagerer, M. 4 case descriptions of boys with the encopresis system. *Prax Kinderpsychol. Kinderpsychiatr.,* 1977, **26**, 21–27.

Wagner, B.R. and Paul, G.L. Reduction of incontinence in chronic mental patients: A pilot project. *Journal of Behavior Therapy and Experimental Psychiatry,* 1970, **1**, 29–38.

Warson, S.R., Caldwell, M.R., Warriner, A., Kirk, A.J. and Jensen, R.A. The dynamics of encopresis. *American Journal of Orthopsychiatry,* 1954, **24**, 402–415.

Watson, L.S. Application of behavior-shaping devices to training severely and profoundly mentally retarded children in an institutional setting. *Mental Retardation,* 1968, **6**, 21–23.

Watts, C. A primary approach to encopresis. *Special Education Forward Trends,* 1977, **4**, 25–26

Weissenberg, S. Uber enkopresis. *Z. Kinderheilk,* 1926, **40**, 674–677.

Whiting, J.M. and Child, I.L. *Child training and personality.* New Haven, Yale Univ. Press, 1953.

Wolters, W.H.G. Encopresis. *Psychotherapy, Psychosomatics,* 1971, **19**, 266–287.

Wolters, W.H.G. A comparative study of behavioral aspects in encopretic children. *Psychotherapy, Psychosomatics,* 1974, **24**, 86–97.

Woodmansey, A.C. Emotion and the motions. *British Journal of Medical Psychology,* 1968, **40**, 207–223.

Woodmansey, A.C. Wetting and soiling. *British Medical Journal,* 1972, **3**, 161–163.

Wright, D.F. and Bunch, G. Parental intervention in the treatment of chronic constipation. *Journal of Behavior Therapy and Experimental Psychiatry,* 1977, **8**, 93–95.

Wright, L. Handling the encopretic child. *Professional Psychology,* 1973, **4**, 137–144.

Wright, L. Outcome of a standardized program for treating psychogenic encopresis. *Professional Psychology,* 1975, **6**, 453–456.

Wright, L. and Walker, C.E. Treatment of a child with psychogenic encopresis. *Clinical Pediatrics,* 1977, **16**, 1042–1045.

Young, G.C. The treatment of childhood encopresis by conditioned gastro-ileal reflex training. *Behavior Research and Therapy,* 1973, **11**, 499–503.

Young, I.L. and Goldsmith, A.O. Treatment of encopresis in a day treatment program. *Psychotherapy: Theory, Research and Practice,* 1972, **9**, 231–235.

Part II
Childhood Enuresis

1

Introduction

HISTORICAL BACKGROUND

After reviewing the history of enuresis, Glicklich (1951) reports that it was initially recognized as a medical problem by the Egyptians in 1550 B.C., and was listed as a distinct disease in the first book of pediatrics written in English in a section entitled "Of Pyssying in the Bedde." Glicklich ended his review with the following conclusion:

> "Enuresis was born with the dawn of civilization and is still with us. Its history is long and colorful with prognosis for a longer and more exciting life before its problems are, if ever, resolved. Basically, enuresis is a symptom, not a disease, and as such it is only with greater understanding of the underlying pathology, be it organic or psychogenic, that we ever hope to conquer it." (p. 874)

Since ancient times a wide variety of folk remedies have been used to eliminate bedwetting, such as raising the foot off the bed, sleeping on the back, drastically restricting fluid intake at bedtime, periodically awakening the child at night to go to the toilet, and consumption of various potions. Among the more inhumane folk remedies used by parents have been tying the penis, placing the buttocks on a hot stove, cold streams of water directed onto the child's lower spine, beating, shaming or ridiculing the child after each bedwetting incident, hitting or threatening severe physical punishment, making the child wear his wet pajamas around his neck or hanging his wet sheets out the window as a means of shaming the child. Smith (1974) reports the case of a child who was brutally burned with a hot poker and threatened by his mother with further mutilation if he continued wetting. Baller (1975) cites the incident where one parent made a 10-year-old boy wear a knotted rope around his waist and sleep in the bathtub. The rope was tied in such a way as to have the knot located in the small of the back in the hope that the discomfort thus produced would prevent the child from sleeping soundly. In a light sleep it was thought that the child would respond to the sensation of a full bladder and awaken in time to avoid wetting. In the 17th century some parents made their enuretic child drink a pint of his own urine.

Parents were not the only ones to engage in various forms of child abuse to "cure" bed wetting. Throughout the ages physicians have treated enuresis with harsh methods and seemed to have little concern with the child's general welfare. In 1500 B.C., doctors were prescribing ground hedgehog and white hyacinthamum flowers for wetting. Hollis Phaer, the father of modern pediatrics, suggested in 1535 the use of the stones of a hedgehog, and other physicians of that day recommended the viscera of pigs and urine of spayed swine. Glicklich (1951) notes that in the 18th century physicians would apply blisters to the sacrum to heat the sacral nerves with a view to making them work more effectively. In the 19th century, mattresses with steel spikes and frames for pelvic elevation were invented. Some practitioners cauterized the child's urethra with silver nitrate. Others inserted rubber bags into a girl's vagina and inflated it with air to compress the bladder neck and urethra.

Fortunately, more effective and humane ways of treating bedwetting have been discovered in recent years although many harsh and abusive methods are still in use today.

DEFINITION

Enuresis was originally derived from the Greek term: I make water. Following customary usage, enuresis is herein defined as "the repeated, involuntary discharge of urine after the age of three years." The age limit of three is chosen because this is the age at which most children achieve urinary continence at night (Powell, 1951). The criterion of *frequent* bedwetting has varied to date. Frequencies of five to seven times a week have been used by some (Agarawala and

Heycock, 1968), while other investigators, such as Epstein and Guilfoyle (1965), stressed that enuresis must be considered a problem by the parents, in addition to a minimal incidence rate of three or so times a week. Clearly, an occasional wet bed at night would not be considered an enuresis problem requiring treatment.

Enuresis has been further classified as nocturnal (nighttime) wetting or diurnal (daytime) wetting; and as primary or secondary. Primary (or essential) enuresis refers to children who never achieved a significant period of dryness, while secondary (or acquired) enuresis refers to children who were dry both day and night for a period of at least six months. Since most of the literature is concerned with nocturnal enuresis or bedwetting, this disorder will be the focus of this section of the book.

Wetting has been found to be nocturnal, only in 60 to 80 percent of enuretic children, diurnal, only in about 5 percent, and nocturnal and diurnal in 20 to 40 percent (Campbell, 1951). Studies to date indicate that when there is both nocturnal and diurnal wetting, then quite good results can be obtained by treating the easier, nighttime wetting; in about half of these cases the daytime enuresis remits spontaneously without having to establish a complex daytime treatment program.

INCIDENCE

It is well known that the incidence of bedwetting declines with the age of the child (Jones, 1960). Chamberlin (1974) found that while 82 percent of middle-class two-year-olds wet the bed at age two, this percentage declines to 49 percent at age three, and 26 percent at age four. Whereas about 20 to 25 percent of four and five-year-olds still bedwet, the number declines to about 10 percent of six to ten year olds, and, finally, to about 3 percent in the teen years and in adulthood (Cushing and Baller, 1976; Wadsworth, 1944; Plag, 1964). It is estimated that between three to seven million schoolage children suffer from this problem in the United States. Thus, the enuretic child should be helped to realize that he or she is not odd or strange because of this problem, that indeed *many* other children are experiencing the same difficulty.

In regard to spontaneous remission of bedwetting, a study of 1129 enuretic children (Forsythe and Redmond, 1974) revealed that the annual spontaneous cure rate for enuretic children between the ages of five and nine years was 14 percent; between 10 and 14 years, 16 percent; and between 15 and 19 years, 19 percent. Three percent of the cases in this long-term follow up study were still wetting after 20 years. It seems that a five-year-old child has only about a 50 percent chance of outgrowing the problem by age ten, and that it may take several years for this remission to happen.

Twice as many boys as girls are generally reported to be enuretic (White, 1971). Also, the incidence in the lower classes is twice that of the middle-class (Bloomfield and Douglas, 1956). The incidence of bedwetting is higher for children placed in the care of others because of the inability of their own families to care for them (Stein and Susser, 1966). Dittman and Blinn (1955) estimate that up to 30 percent of institutionalized youth may wet the bed.

It is clear from the various surveys that about 20 percent of four to five-year-olds still wet the bed with sufficient frequency to constitute a management problem for their parents. Although all but three percent of these children will stop wetting on their own accord by the end of adolescence, there is a need for effective intervention to relieve the burden on the parents, and to forestall difficulties in the child's personality and social development. In answer to the question as to the age when a child's bedwetting should be considered a problem, it usually seems that if a child is still wetting frequently at age five, the parents should seek professional assistance in implementing a treatment program. To wait any longer would be to jeopardize the child's self-esteem, progress in school, and ability to make friends.

CHILD REACTIONS

The reactions of children to their bedwetting vary widely. A common reaction is an outward indifference to the problem. Some children see the wetting as a normal thing that will eventually go away. Others, when asked why they just wet the bed, will attempt to justify the wetting by saying that they've just been to the bathroom. Some children are intensely embarrassed or ashamed of the wetting. They may attempt to run away from the problem by such tactics as becoming deep sleepers; developing a sort of envelope around themselves to keep out things that hurt; or withdrawing from school tasks when they become difficult.

It is noteworthy that many families seem unperturbed about the bedwetting problem in their children and never bring it to professional attention (Freeman, 1975).

ETIOLOGY: UNDERLYING CAUSES OF BEDWETTING

Theories about the underlying causes of enuresis are numerous, and none has been conclusively proven. A few theories have been ruled out however. The ideas that the child does it out of spite/hostility or a way to gain attention, are almost unanimously rejected by professionals in the field. There is just no evidence to support these positions.

Psychological Factors

Emotional Disturbance. Studies show that the incidence of signs of emotional disturbance in enuretic children is about 10 to 15 percent higher than in nonenuretics. It is clear that these signs occur in only a minority of bedwetters, that is, about one in five (Rutter *et al.*, 1973; Taylor and Turner, 1975; Werry, 1967; White, 1971). In the few enuretic children who do show signs of emotional disturbance, it is often not certain if the emotional upset is the effect or the cause of the bedwetting or neither. It is apparent, however, that when the bedwetting is corrected, many of these emotional disturbance signs disappear in a large number of cases (Baller, 1975).

Among the emotional disturbances or behavior difficulties that have been associated with some enuretic children are the following: nail biting, thumb sucking, poor school adjustment, temper tantrums, negativism, firesetting, jealousy of siblings, poor attention span, eating disorders, and stuttering (Benjamin *et al.*, 1971; Despert, 1944; Faschingbauer, 1975).

Fear and anxiety signs have also been evident in some enuretic children. It is well known that fear has a tendency to produce a voiding reaction in humans. Galdston and Perlmutter (1973) found that anxiety in children can alter the frequency and disturb the adequacy of voiding. It is little wonder, then, that children living in areas experiencing frequent bombings during wartime have a higher incidence of bedwetting than usual.

It is also understandable that a recurrence of enuresis in children has been found to be associated with stressful events (Jehu *et al.*, 1977).

A large number of writers have concluded that secondary enuresis is largely a reaction to a stressful or traumatic event in a child's life, such as the birth of a sibling. For instance, Werry (1967) studied 58 cases of secondary enuresis and observed that the "overwhelmingly commonest cause was situational stress," such as hospitalization of the child or separation from the mother.

Apart from increasing the chances of urination, intense anxiety has also been found to impede efficient learning. A high level of anxiety has been found by research to retard new learning and this principle has been termed the Yerkes-Dobson Law (Yerkes and Dobson, 1908). So high anxiety in a child about to be toilet trained could prove inimical to the development of bladder control.

There is some evidence to suggest that as a group enuretic children are more likely to have experienced some environmental stress during the period when children are normally learning urinary continence (Douglas, 1973). Benjamin *et al.* (1971) report that more enuretic children experienced separation from an important child-caring person during the critical age period of two-and-a-half to five years and, thus, have a greater fear of abandonment.

In sum, the evidence to date indicates that the large majority of bedwetting children are not emotionally disturbed. The fact is that four out of five enuretic children seem happy, well adjusted children who wet the bed for other reasons. There is, however, a small group of bedwetting children who show signs of emotional disturbances, and who could probably benefit from counseling or psychotherapy. The child who displays secondary enuresis, that is, relapses after 12 months of being dry at night, seems most likely to be wetting because of anxiety related to environmental stress.

Parental Toilet Training Practices. It has been suggested that if parents pressure a child for nighttime control when the child is not mature enough, the child may lose confidence, become anxious, and thus experience difficulty staying dry at night. Powell (1951) stated that toilet training undertaken at too early an age is conducive to later enuresis. In a study of 41 enuretic children, Bindelglas, Dee, and Enos (1968) found that 35 experienced early toilet training. Furthermore, the parents of 29 of these children admitted that their training was "rigidly strict." Parental rigidity, inconsistency, and frequent use of punishment in toilet training children were found by Despert (1944) as leading to enuresis.

Klackenberg (1955), on the other hand, presented strong evidence that there is no correlation between parental toilet training efforts (either timing or intensity) and the development of enuresis. Benjamin *et al.* (1971) concluded that enuresis is not due to poor training procedures by parents but is related to less frequent use of good training practices. Further research is obviously needed to investigate the relationship, if any, between enuresis and toilet training procedures in the home.

Faulty Learning. Many theorists believe that enuresis is simply a failure by the child to learn to develop adequate cortical control over subcortical reflex mechanisms. Mowrer and Mowrer (1938) stated that the majority of enuretic children wet the bed because they are unable to break the infantile habit of nocturnal reflex voiding. They felt that it is difficult for a child, especially if he is a deep sleeper, to learn to associate the vague sensation of bladder fullness with the response of awakening and contraction of the urethral sphincters. Thus, nighttime voiding continues and becomes such a strong habit that it is very difficult to break.

The fact that mentally retarded children have considerable difficulty learning to control their elimination functions seems to support the idea that this is a difficult learning experience for a child.

Physical Factors

Heredity. Stalker and Rand (1946) list the following constitutional factors that have been linked with enuresis: (1) predominance in males; (2) greater incidence of autonomic disorders such as heavy sleep; (3) a greater number of psychosomatic disorders; and (4) frequent family history of enuresis. A number of studies do report a higher incidence of enuresis, past or present, among the immediate families of enuretic children than among the immediate families of nonenuretics. About 40 to 55 percent of bedwetting children have parents or close relatives who had a similar problem (Abe *et al.*, 1967; White, 1971; Young, 1963). A family history of enuresis is higher for primary than for secondary enuretics. Schauffler (1942) agrees that enuresis does tend to run in families but feels this is due more to environmental influences such as sloppy personal habits. Although a family history of enuresis has been linked with enuretic children, such a history has not been found to seriously affect the likelihood of a prompt recovery with treatment.

Slow Maturation. Many writers support the idea that a large number of wetters suffer from a maturational lag in processes related to effective bladder function. This developmental delay in neurophysiological development may be hereditary. However, facts like occasional dry nights and periods of dryness for bedwetters are hard to reconcile with slow maturation of bladder control mechanisms.

White (1971) believes that enuresis is the result of a developmental lag interacting with maladaptive training practices. He feels that if parents were to completely ignore the slow development of bladder control it would lead to spontaneous cure by the time the child reaches seven or eight years. Unfortunately, he asserts that it is never ignored; 30 percent of the mothers he worked with admitted scolding or beating the child; and those who were not obviously disapproving, made their attitude plain even if they only used the kind words they claimed to use. The results of this, according to White, is that the child becomes anxious and tries very hard to have a dry bed; as he has not yet acquired control, this is impossible and he becomes depressed and the anxiety is reinforced. The effect of anxiety on an enuretic child, as with a child with a stammer, is to make the situation worse rather than better, and a vicious cycle is established. So White (1971) concludes that the cause of bedwetting for many children is a hereditary neuromuscular disability which is aggravated by a child's anxiety over an inability to satisfy parental expectations.

Sleep Arousal Disorders. The question is often raised as to whether bedwetters are inclined to be more deep sleepers than nonbedwetters. In a deep sleep it is felt that a child does not tune in to increased bladder pressure. There have been limited studies and conflicting findings to date in this regard. Many therapists and parents are convinced that the bedwetter is a deep sleeper, but even if this is so, deep sleep may be the result of wetting. Some writers report lighter sleep by wetters after the wetting habit is corrected.

Apart from deep sleep, other sleep arousal disorders such as somnambulism and somniloquy have been associated with enuresis in children (Kales, Jacobson and Kales, 1968; Bakwin, 1970). In this connection, Finley and Wansley (1977) state that the single most important and frequent correlate of enuresis is an elevated arousal threshold during sleep. An elevated arousal threshold is to be distinguished from deep sleep, which is traditionally defined by EEG monitoring of the stages of sleep. Arousal threshold is defined by progressive increments of intensity until the sleeper is awake both behaviorally and electroencephalographically (EEG). Not only is an enuretic child while sleeping, they maintain, relatively unresponsive to internal stimulation such as a distended and rapidly contracting bladder, but also to external stimulation such as a buzzer. Thus, they conclude enuresis is a disorder in the sleep-arousal system. A high intensity alarm seems more likely to penetrate this elevated arousal threshold. They recommend using a 105 dB alarm to start with for the bell and pad apparatus.

Small Bladder Capacity. Difficulty holding urine both during the day and the night has been reported to be associated with enuretic children. It is felt by some that the frequent urination during the day is a sign that some enuretic children empty their bladders in response to very weak distention cues, and thus have a small functional bladder capacity. By training the child to hold his urine at night, this control of the urge to urinate often generalizes to the daytime problem as well (Taylor and Turner, 1975). Muellner (1963) had repeatedly asserted that reduced bladder capacity is a common cause of enuresis in children, and he advocates training children to hold back urination for longer periods so as to increase the capacity.

While the bladder does increase in size with age, it is also a flexible organ that will expand or contract depending upon a number of factors such as the strength of the external sphincter muscles. Also, the bladder contracts with cold, and such factors as being chilled at night may play a role in reducing the functional capacity at night.

It would seem, however, that bladder capacity alone cannot be the sole cause of enuresis because many adults and children with small capacities have diurnal frequency and nocturia, but not enuresis.

Urinary Tract Infection. There is substantial evidence that urinary tract infection is relatively common amongst enuretics. It is even more likely to be present in girls; particularly if they wet the bed every night, where the risk is as high as 1:10 (Taylor and Turner, 1975).

There is no evidence to indicate that the infection is the cause of the enuresis and, actually, the reverse may be true. Galdston and Perlmutter (1973), for example, found that anxiety in children can alter the frequency and disturb the adequacy of voiding to a degree sufficient to dispose the child to urinary tract infection. Also, Forsythe and Redmond (1974) studied 18 enuretic children who had infected urine at the initial exam and found that after treatment of the infection only one child was cured of enuresis. Thus, urinary tract infections seem most likely to be the result not the cause of enuresis. The possibility of an infection should definitely be investigated, however, when the usual accompanying signs are present, such as dysuria, frequency of urination, and often, fever.

Other Organic Factors. A variety of other organic factors have been associated with enuresis, such as:

1. Anatomical defects. Any interference or abnormalities of the nervous system innervating the genito-urinary system can result in enuresis. Such disorders include spinal cord defects, nervous system developmental disorders, and atony of the external sphincter muscle due to an imbalance of the parasympathetic nervous system. An obstruction of the posterior urethral valves can result in difficult or hesitant micturition, urinary frequency and dribbling since birth. Noteworthy is the fact that there are usually other symptoms present with anatomical defects, such as difficulty starting and stopping urination, painful urination, or excessive frequency.

2. Constipation. A large fecal mass can decrease bladder capacity and can trigger long-lasting disorders of bladder control. The use of enemas to relieve the bowel impaction often alleviates the bladder problem.

3. Allergy. An allergy could be the cause since there is some evidence showing that the incidence of bedwetting is much higher in females with allergic disorders than in those without (Gerrard, 1971). This could be because the mucosal lining of the bladder resembles the lining of the respiratory tract and thus might also be vulnerable to allergens.

Most investigators report that the incidence of organic or physiological difficulties resulting in bedwetting is low, that is, these factors seem to account for only 1 to 3 percent of all bedwetters (Baller, 1975; Forsythe and Redmond, 1974). A careful history taking, physical exam, and urinalysis can, in most cases, reveal the presence of organic factors. If there is no evidence of organic involvement, the enuresis should be classified as psychogenic and treated accordingly.

Summary and Conclusions

A review of the literature leads to the conclusion that no single factor accounts for enuresis, instead, it has a multiple of causes and correlates. No one variable seems to be a very strong predictor. The disorder appears to arise from a combination of a number of factors which interrelate in various ways with one another and which differ from one child to another.

It is clear that organic factors by themselves give rise to a *very small proportion* of enuretic cases. Since enuresis is primarily psychogenic in origin, then, it should be considered a psychosomatic disorder rather than a disease.

PHYSIOLOGY OF THE URINARY SYSTEM

Urine is continually discharged from the kidneys and enters the upper end of the bladder by means of two small ducts called ureters.

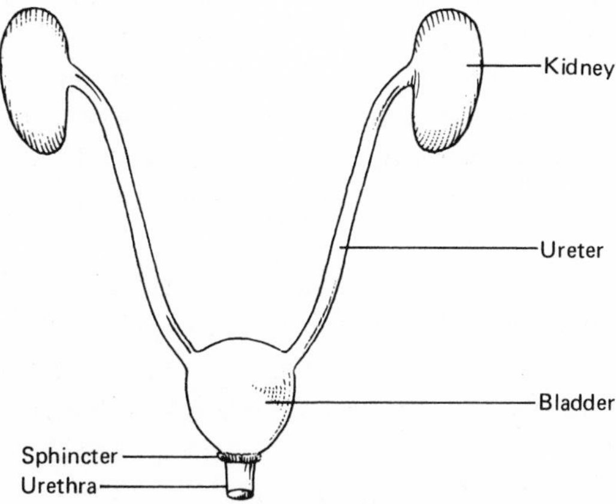

Figure 3. Diagram of Urinary System.

The mouth of each ureter, where it enters the bladder, serves as a valve to prevent a backflow of urine into the ureter when the bladder pressure increases. The bladder functions as a storage bag for the urine and it expands to a certain point and then its muscles contract to discharge the urine into the tube at its lower end called the urethra (See Figure 3). The round bands of muscles that close the entrance to the urethra are called sphincters. Urine is retained in the bladder by two ring-shaped muscles which encircle the urethra and the neck of the bladder, and whose contraction keeps the bladder outlet closed. The opening of the internal sphincter is due to contraction of involuntary muscles of the bladder, while the external sphincter muscle is under voluntary control. The muscle that enables one to start and stop the flow of urine is the external sphincter.

The outer layer of the bladder wall contains circular bands of muscles called detrusor muscles whose contractions squeeze the bladder and increase bladder pressure. The degree of bladder pressure also depends upon the amount of accumulated urine in the bladder. The bladder muscles do not contract unless they receive nervous impulses, set in motion by the stimulation of sense organs in the bladder wall when the bladder is distended.

The micturitional reflex consists of a strong contraction of the detrusor muscles and relaxation of the internal sphincter, followed by relaxation of the external sphincter. There is a reciprocally inhibitory relationship between the detrusor and the internal sphincter. When the internal sphincter muscle, located at the neck of the bladder relaxes, urine is allowed to pass into the first third of the urethra. The final barrier, the external sphincter muscle, is located here. Although under voluntary control, the external sphincter tends to relax in response to bladder pressure and to the flow of urine as it passes the first sphincter. When both sphincters are relaxed, voiding occurs.

In the infant, micturition is an automatic reflex when the bladder is distended. The muscle wall of the bladder rounds out and stretches as urine accumulates. Stretch receptors in these detrusor muscles send neural impulses to the spinal cord via the pelvic nerve. A reflex arc in the spinal cord sends parasympathetic impulses back down the pelvic nerve causing the muscle wall to contract. This upsets the balance between the bladder's contents, opening the internal sphincter slightly. A small amount of urine enters the urethra and activates sensors there which in turn signal the spinal cord. A reflex arc in the spinal cord sends motor impulses back which open the external sphincter permitting urination. The process continues until the urethra is void of urine. Then the sphincters close, stopping the process.

The normal child is able to inhibit urination beyond the point of the first sensations of urgency, and to initiate micturition at low bladder pressures. The child gains cortical control of the detrusor as a result of maturation and learned associations. Also, in voluntary micturition, the detrusor is induced to contract by contracting the lower abdominal muscles, and by relaxing the pelvic floor muscles. This action results in a rapid lowering of the bladder neck and the descent of the neck provides the stimulus for detrusor contraction. Holding of urine is apparently achieved by the opposite maneuver, helped along by crossing one's legs or holding one's groin.

Normally, daytime control of the bladder transfers to the sleeping state. This control, together with the reduced flow of urine during the night, allows the child to sleep through the night.

The amount of urine delivered by the kidneys at any given time depends upon a number of factors, such as the amount of fluids and solids consumed, the temperature and humidity of the air, the amount of muscular exercise, and emotional stress. The more rapidly the bladder fills, the more sensitive the neural mechanism is to bladder pressure, and the greater is the feeling of urgency. When the bladder fills slowly, a considerable amount of pressure can be tolerated.

A state of alarm tends to reduce the flow of urine from the kidneys, and to shift water from the blood to the tissues. A state of dread or intense fear, however, also may lessen the output of urine, but it produces a tendency towards bladder spasm and sphincter release that is somewhat independent of bladder volume. As a result, intense anxiety in children (as in wartime) results in an increased incidence of enuresis. Both the absorption of water by the body, and the voiding of urine are adaptive strategies to danger since they prepare the body for strenuous exercise.

Functional Bladder Capacity

In the normal three-to-four-year-old child the desire to micturate occurs after about 100 mls. (3.5 ounces) of urine have been slowly introduced into the bladder, and this is termed the average functional bladder capacity (Doleys and Wells, 1975). When maximum bladder capacity is reached (about 7 ounces for most children) an intense desire to micturate occurs and emptying becomes essential. The average adult bladder can hold 500 ml but the urge to go is present at about 200–350 ml. Studies by Zaleski, Gerrard and Shokeir (1973) have suggested that enuretic children have smaller maximum bladder capacities, compared to nonenuretics. Also, they have shown that increased bladder capacity seems to occur in children who respond to drug and dietary treatments. It would seem reasonable to conclude that similar changes accompany successful bell and pad treatment methods.

Braithwaite (1956) found that the bladders of many enuretic children contracted after the introduction of only small volumes of fluids. All but 4 of the 117 children studied desired to micturate with less than 100 mls, and 58 with less than 10 mls. This suggests a failure of the detrusor muscle to relax. Similarly, Broughton (1968) presented evidence that spontaneous bladder contractions are more frequent and powerful in enuretic children and that some of these contractions culminate in wetting incidents. Also noteworthy is the finding by DiPerry and Medurri (1972) that artificial filling of the bladder in sleeping children produced reflex urination in enuretic children whereas it produced arousal without wetting in nonenuretic children.

McLellan (1939) described two types of abnormal bladder function in severely enuretic children: uninhibited rhythmic contractions of the detrusor muscles occurring after the introduction of 25–75 mls. fluid, increasing in intensity until the bladder is filled; or a smooth rise in pressure until bladder filling was completed and then there was an imperative need to empty. Finally, Muellner (1963) demonstrated by X-ray studies that the bladder in enuretic children is small, and he suggested that this is due to the failure of the enuretic child to fully master voluntary control over the act of micturition.

It would seem from the above studies that a number of enuretic children have difficulty inhibiting their bladder-emptying mechanisms and that this difficulty plays a major role in their enuresis.

2

Toilet Training Practices and Childhood Enuresis

Toilet training problems are still a major concern of American parents according to the results of a recent survey (Mesibov *et al.*, 1977). Next to disobedience and whining this was the biggest concern the parents expressed about raising children.

Control of the bowel is achieved by the average child by 18 to 24 months of age. Daytime control of the bladder is accomplished by almost all children by the age of four years, and control at night by four-and-a-half years. As previously mentioned, girls tend to be ahead of boys in respect to both bowel and bladder control. In the typical sequence, children first acquire control of the bowel asleep, then control of the bowel awake, then control of the bladder awake, and then, after a rather variable interval, control of the bladder while asleep at night. Children delayed in one aspect of sphincter development tend to be delayed in the others. Children are born with reflex voiding reactions. The bladder fills and the infant voids automatically. During the years one to three, the nerve pathways that transmit information from the brain to the bladder develop so that cognitive control over the bladder increases. Nighttime wetting occurs when daytime control has been established, because it is more difficult to control the natural tendency to void when one is asleep and has diminished cognitive and conscious control of bodily processes.

According to Despert (1944), parents can expect daytime control by age two-and-a-half, and nighttime control by three years. The average age the children in her study achieved daytime bladder control was 21 months; night control at 27 months. The average age training was begun was 2.8 months.

Progress in bladder training is slow until age 24 months, when the child responds well to praise and verbalizes his/her needs. At age 30 months, urine retention lasts about five hours. By 36 months the child may stay dry throughout the night, although occasional accidents can be expected through age five years. Between ages five and eight bedwetting will occur only rarely, such as after an exciting day, a cold night or a frightening TV program.

Studies have shown that, in general, children under 24 months of age require more training time to achieve full control of their bowels and bladders (Matson and Ollendick, 1977). Azrin and Foxx (1974) and Butler (1976) found that children over 25 to 26 months of age were toilet trained in about half the time as younger children, and that girls trained somewhat faster than boys.

The difference between boys and girls in acquiring control, and evidence relating enuresis to retarded skeletal maturity, links enuresis to the rate of physical maturation and sphincter development (Stein and Susser, 1967).

EFFECTIVE BLADDER TRAINING

Benjamin *et al.* (1971 a, b) conducted a survey to identify the toilet training practices employed by parents who had no problem training their children. The following procedures were found to be effective:

1. Use cues and prompts. For example, switch from diapers at night to training pants or pajamas.
2. Try to wait until it is the child's idea that it is time to start night training. Wait until a child feels a sense of responsibility for accidents at night, and shows a concern about nighttime wetting.
3. When a child wakes up dry in the morning pick him up, kiss and hug him. Say in a pleased manner, "You can keep dry pants all by yourself."
4. Have the child urinate just before bed and immediately upon arising in the morning.
5. Parents should have the expectation that the child will not need to urinate at all during the night.
6. When the child wakes up wet early in the training say, "Don't worry, let's try to do better next time."

Benjamin *et al.* (1971) note that it is not helpful to restrict fluids at night, wake the child up to urinate just before the parents retire, or to stop the night bottle. It is also not beneficial to give a concrete reward, such as a toy, for a dry night. Also, the following comments impede the training: "Shame on you, you naughty boy." "You are just lazy and dirty." "I don't like you when you wet at night."

Most writers recommend a similar common sense strategy involving such key elements as:

1. Waiting until the child shows signs of readiness (dry naps, awareness of being wet and desire to be dry.
2. Giving positive reinforcement for dry nights by praise and attention.
3. Prompting the child that you expect nighttime dryness now. Switch to training pants at night. Do not keep a child in diapers at night when he/she is seven, eight, and nine years old. This is counterproductive. Signal the child that you believe bladder control at night is now possible and expected.
4. Being patient and understanding. Expect accidents to happen occasionally.
5. Not using power-related strategies such as shaming, threats, or punishment for failures.

Litrownik (1974) stated that, in general, effective toilet training involves three steps: In the first, habit training, the child is placed on the toilet and any eliminative effort or response is reinforced by parental attention or other rewards. A number of prompts, such as verbal instructions or demonstrations may be employed in an attempt to initiate the desired response on the part of the child. After a number of practice sessions the child learns to respond appropriately when the parents place him or her on the toilet, but "accidents" may still occur. In the second stage the child begins to "inform" the parents either verbally or nonverbally when elimination is anticipated. The parents respond to this cue by either taking the child to the bathroom, or directing the child to "go to the bathroom." The final step usually involves a gradual unsystematic fading of parent intervention resulting in independent toileting behavior on the part of the child.

Most children go through these steps, in varying lengths of time, with little or no problem. But in approximately 10 percent of the population, especially with lower IQ children, extreme difficulty due to inadequate training methods is experienced (Werry, 1967).

For these hard-to-train children a more intensive program seems needed.

Brazelton (1962) recommends a child-oriented approach to toilet training which involves a relaxed, unpressured approach by the parents, and only starting training when the child shows a physical and psychological readiness to cooperate. More specifically, the procedure is as follows: Some time after the child is 18 months old, a "potty chair" on the floor is introduced as the child's own chair. The parents verbally associate it with the parents' toilet seat. At some routine time, the parents take the child each day to sit on the chair in all his clothes (least the unfamiliar feeling of a cold seat impede progress). At this time, the parent sits with him, reads to him or gives him a cookie. Since he is sitting on a chair on the floor, he is free to leave at will. There should never be any coercion or pressure to remain on the seat. After a week or so of the child's cooperation in this part of the procedure, he can be taken with his diapers off, to sit on the chair for another period. Still no attempt to "catch" his stool or urine is made. This gradual introduction to the chair avoids frightening him or giving him the feeling he is "losing part of himself" by eliminating in the chair.

After the above steps are achieved the child can be taken to the pot a second time during the day. This can be after his diapers are soiled to change him on the seat, dropping his dirty diaper under him into the pot and explaining to him that this is the eventual function of his chair.

When the child shows some understanding of the chair's purpose and a wish to comply, he can be taken several times a day to "catch" his urine or stool. As his interest grows, all diapers and pants are removed for short periods and the potty chair is placed in his play area or nearby and his ability to go on his own is pointed out. He is urged to go to the pot by himself when he wishes. He may be reminded of this periodically during the day. Training pants can be introduced at this point. Children often show excitement at the ability to master these steps. Only after the child has mastered daytime control is nap and night training introduced. This may be one to two years later.

Brazelton reports that daytime training is completed between two and two and one-half years for 80 percent of the children trained by the above procedure. Night training was accomplished by three years in 80 percent of the cases. Males and first-born children took longer to complete the training.

Spock and Bergen (1964) recommend looking for signs of readiness in a child 18 to 24 months of age, and then tactfully asking for his cooperation until success is achieved. Among the readiness signs one might look for in regard to bowel control are the ability to walk, pull down training pants, some degree of regularity in elimination, and signs of discomfort or displeasure following soiling. Signs of bladder readiness usually appear between ages two and one-half to three years and include the achievement of bowel control, being dry for at least two-hour periods during the day, waking up dry from naps, and signs of displeasure or discomfort at being wet.

After reviewing the literature, Walker (1978) suggests the following procedures for toilet training a child:

1. Allow child to observe other family members toileting and encourage him to do the same.
2. Recognize and give mild praise for any signs of cooperation or success by the child and label it an indication of becoming a grown-up person.
3. If the above steps fail to produce any response the child is probably not ready, so training should be postponed while showing no signs of displeasure. After waiting two to three months make another attempt to train.
4. Give the training in a relatively low-key, matter-of-fact way with an underlying expression of confidence in the child's ability to be successful when ready.
5. If a child is not trained by age five, a more rigorous approach should be used, such as the Azrin and Foxx rapid training method.

Among the pitfalls to avoid while toilet training are the following (Homan, 1977):

Do not leave the child on the toilet for long periods of time.

Do not play with the child on the toilet.

Do not give excessive praise for success on the chair.

Do not show disgust at sight of bowel movements.

Do not put on chair if child cries at the experience.

Do not try to train while the child is sick, out of sorts, is being taught other lessons in behavior, or is under stress because of a recent trauma or changes in the home environment.

Do not leave the child alone on the toilet in the early stages of training.

By way of a review and summary of effective toilet training procedures, the following positive and negative practices are presented:

Accentuate the Positives

1. *Do* teach children words to signal the need to eliminate ("Go potty" Make a duty"). Keep repeating the words in the proper context so they become part of the child's vocabulary.

2. *Do* provide a potty chair for toilet training. Make the child feel it is his or her own possession. A potty chair is better than an adult toilet because the child can plant his/her own feet firmly on the floor, is more comfortable in a seat his/her own size, and is less fearful of falling in a low chair. Inform the child that the potty is to be used in the same way as your toilet.

3. *Do* praise the child for sitting on the potty and for any elimination successes. Provide other incentives for sitting such as toys and books to be used *only* when on the potty. Give an immediate food reward (nuts, dried fruit, cookies) for an elimination on the potty. Do set up a star chart to mark a child's progress and to provide special rewards for clean pants or dry nights. Praise the child for progress in front of other family members.

4. *Do* increase a child's motivation for toilet training by associating it with "being grown up" and with being comfortably clean. Review with the child the inconveniences associated with wetting and soiling.

5. *Do* give the child the sense that toilet training is really his or her own responsibility. Consider waiting until the child seems eager to be trained, and willing to take an active role in the process.

6. *Do* establish a schedule and toilet the child at regular times each day, such as after meals, before and after naps, and once or twice in between. Give the child verbal encouragement to use the potty at these times.

7. *Do* try to "anticipate" elimination, that is, observe the child for early signs of the need to go, such as squirming, grunting, and

different facial expressions. Take the child to the toilet when these signs are evident. Praise any successes and point out to the child that he or she should voluntarily go to the bathroom when such urges occur.

8. *Do* give gentle reminders to use the potty during the early stages of toilet training. In other words, ask the child at regular intervals if he/she has to go.

9. *Do* switch to training pants rather than diapers to signal the child that you believe he or she is ready to control these functions. Let the child know how proud you are that he/she has graduated to this stage of maturity.

10. *Do* show the child that you expect him/her to become successful in using the potty every time he/she feels to need to go.

11. *Do* allow the child to observe other family members using the toilet appropriately. Children learn a great deal by observing and imitating others.

12. *Do* postpone training if a child does not seem ready or resists training efforts.

13. *Do* call a child in from play to use the bathroom if he/she frequently has accidents during playtime. Let the child know that when he/she can come in by him/herself you won't have to call.

14. *Do* look for signs that a child is ready for training, such as not soiling at night, waking up dry from a two-hour nap, seems aware of own eliminations, or seems uncomfortable when dirty.

15. *Do* not begin training too early. Remember that the later one initiates bowel training, the shorter the time required to complete the training. Thus, after 20 to 24 months of age, children need less time to achieve success.

16. *Do* expect children to have some "accidents" even after they seem almost trained. It is best to either ignore these accidents or to just give a mild reprimand such as, "I'm disappointed that you forgot to use the potty."

17. *Do* remain calm, patient, and understanding during the training process. Expect gradual progress rather than instant success.

Give constant encouragement and very little discipline. Use positive methods of training (praise, rewards, reassurance, and positive expectancy of success) rather than negative methods (yelling, punishing).

18. *Do* strive for a middle ground between being too lenient/lax and being too strict/punitive in your toilet training.

19. *Do* remember that it is unlikely that children wet or soil because they are lazy, obstinate, or rebellious. Accidents are much more likely to be due to slow physiological development, insecurity-anxiety, or ignoring signals due to intense involvement in play or other tasks.

20. *Do* remember that toilet training difficulty is a common problem in childhood and is usually not a sign of deep seated personality problems in the child.

Minimize the Negatives

1. *Do not* use harsh punishments when a child has an accident. Spanking or hitting a child tend to make the problem worse.

2. *Do not* use such negative tactics as blaming, shaming, threatening, moralizing, or name calling. These methods tend to exacerbate the problem by making the child nervous, embarrassed, resentful, and unhappy. Examples of such methods are: "For shame!" "You're going to be very sorry if you dirty your pants again." "Bad boy!" "What a baby you are!" "That's disgusting!" "If you loved me you'd stop that wetting." "You're just lazy and don't care." "What's the matter with you?"

3. *Do not* insist that the child remain on the potty for more than 5 to 10 minutes. However, do not read to the child or let him play with the bathroom toys if he gets off the potty seat.

4. *Do not* restrict fluids just before bedtime. This can compound the problem by inducing bladder neck irritation and the urge to micturate at lower than normal volumes of bladder pressure.

5. *Do not* worry if your child is later than other children in achieving bowel or bladder control. Each child develops according to his or her own schedule. Do not try to compete with other families to see who can toilet train their children the earliest.

6. *Do not* worry about night training once a child is trained during the day. Most children just naturally become dry at night when their bladders become mature enough, provided they are not nervous or rebellious. Praise and share in the child's pride when he or she begins to have dry nights.

Instant potty training is still the American dream (Olness, 1977). Thus, considerable interest has been generated by the rapid toilet training method developed by Azrin and Foxx and described in their book *Toilet Training in Less than a Day* (Azrin and Foxx, 1974). Matson (1975) and Butler (1976) report that a number of parents are unsuccessful in training their children if they just read the book; they need close supervision by professionals to be most effective. Even with close supervision, parents can expect their children to exhibit a number of emotional side effects to this intensive treatment, consisting primarily of temper tantrums and avoidance behaviors. These negative reactions were most often in response to the positive practice procedure and the graduated guidance required to keep their children on the potty. Since Azrin and Foxx (1974) used various forms of punishment, such as overcorrection, it should probably be reserved for difficult-to-train children who do not respond to more positive approaches. In the positive approach the child is praised for successes and failures are ignored. Every effort is made to keep the toileting experience as relaxed and pleasant as possible. The use of punishment, scolding, shaming, ridicule, and threats is avoided.

3

Treatment Approaches for Enuresis

In view of the multiple factors associated with the etiology of bedwetting, it is not surprising that there are currently available a wide variety of treatment methods. The major treatment interventions will be discussed in this chapter, beginning with the behavioral conditioning approach which has proved most successful over the years. Other interventions included in this chapter are retention training, periodic awakening, hypnosis, psychodynamic, and drug approaches.

BELL AND PAD CONDITIONING METHOD

For the past 30 years the electric conditioning apparatus, commonly known as the "bell and pad," has gained in popularity and has proven consistently effective. It is the most extensively researched treatment procedure for enuresis, and the one with the best record of initial and lasting success. Thus, the bell and pad is currently the treatment of choice for the majority of enuretic children.

The bell and pad procedure, or urine alarm, was popularized by Mowrer and Mowrer (1938), although Pfaundler (1904) had initially discovered its therapeutic potential. Modifications have been made in the Mowrer-type conditioning instrument over the years to improve its effectiveness. Basically, the apparatus includes a urine-sensitive pad, upon which the child sleeps and activates a loud bell or buzzer when urine passes into the bed. Urine which contains salt and is an electrolyte, completes an electrical circuit in a pad placed under the bottom sheet. The child is awakened by the noise, closes the bladder outlet so as to cease voiding, turns off the alarm, and then completes the act of micturition in the toilet. After this sequence has occurred several times, the child learns the habit of awakening himself to the stimulus of bladder pressure or learns to sleep through the night without losing control of the sphincter muscle. The exact physiological changes occurring as the result of this treatment are not known.

Apparatus

In 1904, Pfaundler constructed a device consisting of two pieces of wire screen separated by cloth connected to batteries and an electric bell. By using this device continuously under a child for a month or so, he found the ringing of the bell had therapeutic effects for enuretic children. Genouville (1908) reported equally good results with this method. The procedure was largely ignored, however, until Mowrer and Mowrer (1938) used a similar device to eliminate enuresis in 30 children ranging in age from 3 to 13 years.

The Mowrer device consists of two wire mesh or aluminum foil pads separated by a gauze pad. Positive and negative wires run from a battery or transformer and are connected to either of the two pads. Leads from either pad run to the positive and negative poles of a bell or buzzer. The pad unit is placed under the sleeping child and is activated when urine seeping through the gauze pads completes the circuit and rings the alarm. The current is too weak to be dangerous or even to be perceptible. In this way, the child is awakened just after the onset of urination.

The pads in the early devices tended to become odorous after use and had to be replaced. In 1936, Seiger (1952) improved the apparatus by incorporating a relay in the electrical circuit which made the device more sensitive and thus more quickly responsive to urine. He also constructed a rectangular rubber pad into which metal strips had been bonded. The metal is bonded flush with the rubber and presents a smooth, flexible, and nonodorous surface. Since the rubber pad only requires one top sheet to be penetrated by the urine as compared with at least two sheets in the use of the wire screen pad, tests have shown that the rubber activates the alarm in one half the time.

The Seiger-type pad is connected to a unit box, and electricity to operate the unit is typically derived from 110 volt AC house current with a transformer to reduce the voltage to safe limits. A drawing of the Seiger apparatus is presented in Figure 4.

The device incorporates both a light and a bell as stimulus to wake the child. The rubber pad can easily be wiped dry after it is damped with urine and is thus immediately reuseable.

In 1965, Coote developed a pad in which the electrodes are recessed below the upper surface, thus precluding the possibility of electricity coming in direct contact with the child's skin. In this way, there is no chance of skin sores or ulcers developing, and there is also little problem of corrosion of the electrodes, or false alarms. This apparatus is, however, more expensive.

It is important to look for high quality equipment that is sensitive to small amounts of urine, is durable and reliable, completely safe from shock or electrochemical burns, and unlikely to produce false alarms. At the present time, there are several sources of equipment. The least expensive are the ones available from the large department

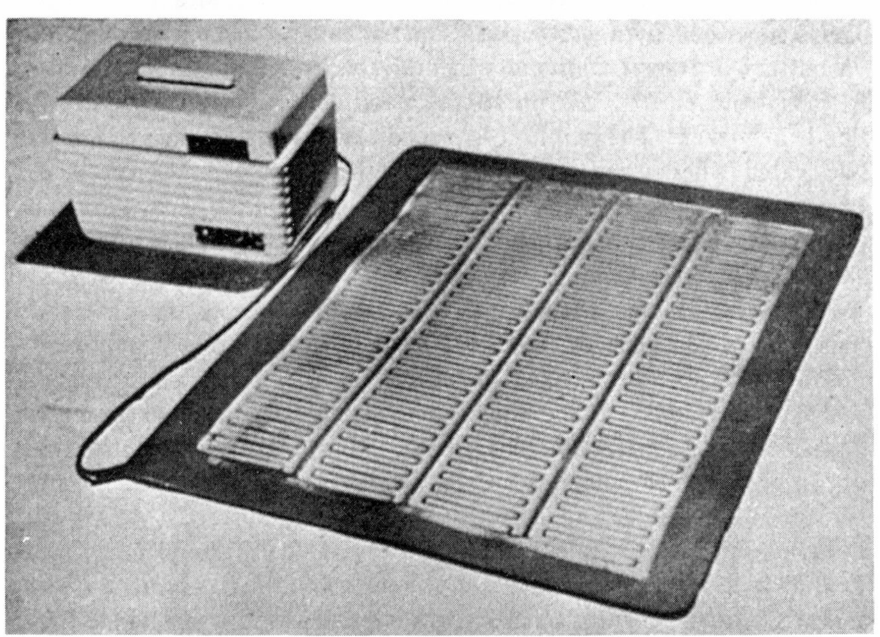

Figure 4. Seiger-type Apparatus for Enuresis.

stores which sell for well under $100. Unfortunately, this equipment has been found to be somewhat unreliable in the past and no supervision is available.

Other sources of bell and pad equipment are the commercial companies that rent equipment and provide supervision. To a large degree, the equipment of the commercial companies appear to be comparable (Doleys, 1977).

Some companies will rent or sell equipment to professional child therapists who can then provide close, personal supervision. Results show that when parents buy equipment and try to train an enuretic child by themselves, they often fail. There is a need for a well trained and experienced child therapist to supervise the training. A listing of such companies can be obtained by writing the author.

Regardless of the device employed, the goal is the same; namely, to immediately condition the inhibition of urination and/or a waking response to threshold bladder pressure. A great advantage of the bell and pad apparatus is that the child does not continue to lie in a wet bed; rather, the child must arise and awaken so that he or she is not allowed to remain indifferent to the problem.

Rationale

Despite much debate, psychologists are still not certain what accounts for the success of the bell and pad. It has been assumed that the apparatus is based on classical conditioning principles, but it has not been found to work in this manner. The idea is that the noise of the buzzer (unconditioned stimulus) trains the child to wake up and pay more attention to the cue of a distended bladder. In this way the child is conditioned to wake up and empty his bladder in the night. But what usually happens is that when children using the bell and pad become dry, they do not wake up and empty their bladders at night, they sleep through quite dry until morning (White, 1971).

Thus, the behavior conditioning seems to work on operant principles, that is, the child learns to associate nocturnal voiding with unpleasant consequences (bell ringing and awakening) so to avoid this, he learns to strengthen his sphincter muscles so he can sleep through the night (Azrin, Sneed and Foxx, 1974).

Stages in Conditioned Response Therapy

Children typically go through the following four steps in the bell and pad conditioning:

In step one, the child continues to urinate with the same or increased frequency as before. Some of the wet spots will become smaller and the frequency of wetting may decrease towards the end of this phase. During the second step, the average size of the wet spots will be smaller, often no more than a few inches in diameter. The frequency of wetting will decrease and the first alarm will ring at a later hour than before. Toward the end of this period the child may "beat the bell" for the first time and awaken to void before actually wetting the bed. During step three, the child awakens before wetting with greater and greater frequency, and finally no longer wets the bed. The child still awakens one or two times to urinate, and still sleeps with the conditioning unit in place. During the fourth and final step, the child sleeps without the conditioning unit. The child will sleep for longer and longer periods between awakening and usually sleeps the whole night without awakening. This final step may vary in length from a few weeks to several months.

Practical Treatment Procedures

The procedure for the use of the bell and pad apparatus is typically as follows:

1. Thoroughly explain to the child and the parents the treatment rationale, the probability of success, the length of treatment, and the possibility of relapse. Attempt to explain the principles of the method in simple terms. Compare the apparatus to a "teaching machine" or "helper" like other home appliances. The instruction to the family should stress child "self-help" under parental supervision. Emphasize the importance of being consistent in the treatment and never skipping a night during the conditioning. Establish rapport with the child and the parents and generate an expectancy of success. Secure a medical exam if there is daytime enuresis to rule out organic factors.

2. Since treatment usually takes two to four months, do not start the conditioning if the family anticipates any interruptions due to vacations, hospitalizations, family moves, etc.

3. For two weeks prior to treatment, a record should be kept, preferably by the child, of bedwetting incidents. A baseline record of nightly incidents enables the therapist to assess treatment progress. Once the baseline recording is started, all other forms of treatment (restriction of fluids, nightly awakening) must be stopped.

4. Make an agreement with the family about the period of time the apparatus will be used after the first dry night is attained. It seems best if the following criterion of success is used: 28 consecutive dry nights with only one accident.

5. Demonstrate the apparatus to the child and the parents. Trigger the alarm by using a saline solution, or metal object such as a spoon or paper clip. Repeat this demonstration with the child holding one hand on the pad so as to be sure there is no shock and nothing to fear.

6. Show the family how to place the pad on the bed. Position the pad on top of a rubber or plastic sheet where the child's buttocks will rest. The long edges of the pad should be parallel with the foot of the bed. The Seiger-type pad is placed on the bed with the metal elements up, and the top of the pad is covered with a sheet or dry diaper. The child sleeps with his/her buttocks resting on the covered pad. Only the top part of the pajamas are worn—the buttocks should be bare.

7. Each night before the child retires the parents and the child are to rehearse the following procedure at least five times. The child lies on the bed and says, "If the bell rings I will get right up." The parents or child should trigger the bell by placing a metal object, such as a key, on the pad. The child then gets right up and turns off the alarm switch. The child should then go to the bathroom and turn the light switch on and off. Then the child returns to the bed and resets the alarm. During the last rehearsal the child should be encouraged to urinate in the toilet. This type of behavior rehearsal helps the child establish the habit of immediately arising once the bell rings, and going to the toilet.

8. When the bell rings at night the child is to get right up and turn off the bell and go to the bathroom to finish voiding. The parent is to be sure the child gets up, and the parent changes the wet sheet while the child is in the bathroom. The parent also fills out the progress report before retiring. The record sheet should specify the date, time, size of the wet spot in inches, and whether the child

awoke to void on his own and, thus, "beat the alarm" (See Table 2). The pad is wiped off by a dry edge of the wet sheet and a dry sheet is placed on the pad. It is important to be sure the child is *thoroughly awakened* by the bell. Turn on the room light when you enter and have the child wash his face to ensure he is awake. The alarm should not be turned off until the child is awake enough to turn it off by himself. The child resets the alarm before going to bed again.

9. During treatment there should be no reduction in the child's normal drinking habits or natural fluid intake. On the contrary, therapists often recommend that during the first two weeks of conditioning the bedwetter be given a glass of water before retiring to increase the frequency of wetting. The more the alarm rings, the more effective the conditioning and the sooner the child will be dry at night.

10. Close supervision by a therapist is important when parents use the bell and pad (Dische, 1973; Lovibond, 1964). The parents should be advised to call the therapist about any difficulty or uncertainty on their part. In addition to regular office visits, the procedure should be monitored by telephone several times a week.

Effectiveness of the Bell and Pad Procedure

About 8 to 12 weeks is the average time for success, but it is quite variable; some children cease wetting almost immediately, and others require over seven months of the conditioning treatment. A recent review of bell and pad studies (Doleys, 1977) indicates that the apparatus is initially effective in arresting bedwetting in 75 percent of the cases, with a relapse rate of about 41 percent. Most of the relapses occurred within six months of treatment, and reapplication of the bell and pad resulted in a 68 percent success rate with the relapse cases. Comparative studies have shown it to be superior to most other forms of treatment. DeLeon and Mandell (1966), for example, compared bell and pad conditioning and psychotherapy in the treatment of enuretic children. They reported cures in 83 percent of the conditioned subjects, 18 percent of the psychotherapy subjects, and 11 percent of the control subjects who received no treatment.

The conditioning method has been found to be useful with diverse populations, such as the mentally retarded, teenagers, and institutionalized children (Jehu *et al.* 1977). Long-term follow up studies

Table 2. Sample Record Form.

Progess Report

Name ______________________________ Age _____

Date	Time	Size of Spot (Diameter in inches) or Beat Alarm	Bedtime	Morning Awake Time	Comments
Example: 5/2/79	10:30	5 inches; 3:30 2 inch	9:00	7:30	10:30 deep sleep

are also favorable. In a 12-year follow-up (Baller and Schalock, 1956), for instance, it was found that dryness was largely sustained throughout the 12-year period by at least 77 percent of the children. Also noteworthy is the fact that no symptom substitution has been found to occur after the bedwetting is eliminated. So the bell and pad has been consistently found to be a robust treatment approach, and has thus become the method of choice for most enuretic cases.

Relapse Rates

Studies show that about 30 to 40 percent of the children relapse after initially becoming dry with the bell and pad procedure. A generally accepted criterion of relapse is a return to regular weekly wetting. This is obviously different from an occasional accident or sporadic wetting. DeLeon and Mandell (1966) report that the severity of relapse is low, and retraining with the apparatus is relatively rapid. Most of the relapses occur within six months of treatment, and it is very rare for a relapse to occur if the child is still dry one year after treatment (Taylor and Turner, 1975).

Overlearning has been reported to be effective in reducing the relapse rate to 20 percent or less. According to Young and Morgan (1972b), the overlearning procedure involves two requirements. First, the conditioning training is extended from the usual success criterion of 14 dry nights to another 14 dry nights. Thus, the child must go 28 consecutive dry nights before the treatment is stopped. The other requirement is that for the extended time period the child must drink a greatly increased amount of liquid (two pints in this study) during the hour just before going to bed. This is presumed to strengthen the ability of the bladder control mechanism to hold urine at night. So lengthening the treatment time and making it more difficult is essentially the overlearning process—a process which has been found to offer an extra assurance of a lasting effect. Taylor and Turner (1975) report that the overlearning procedure brought the relapse rate from 69 percent to 23 percent. They continued treatment until there was no more than one wetting incident in 28 consecutive nights. Also, as soon as the child achieved seven consecutive dry nights, fluid intake was increased by 1-2 pints (according to the child's tolerance).

In addition, Doleys (1977) notes that the use of an intermittent schedule for the alarm, that is, the alarm is set to go off only some of the time after wetting, rather than a continuous schedule, has resulted in a lower relapse rate.

In conclusion, a relatively high relapse rate for the bell and pad has been a problem in the past, and further research is needed in this area. The overlearning procedure seems a particularly promising approach to reducing this difficulty.

Other Problems with Bell and Pad

Apart from the relapse rate, some of the common problems therapists experience in using the conditioning approach are as follows:

1. Lack of Parental Cooperation. According to Doleys (1977), the single most common reason for failure with the urine alarm has been lack of parental cooperation. Many parents have a basic distrust of technology, while others find the two or three months of training too difficult and drop out. Better instruction and closer supervision of the parents have been associated with more successful treatment (Werry and Cohrssen, 1965). It seems, then, that the bell and pad treatment is more likely to succeed if the parents understand how it works and have professional advice and support during treatment. A parents' manual or book explaining the procedure is also very helpful.

2. Child Does not Awaken to Alarm. Another common cause of failure with the bell and pad is the child not waking until the bed is already thoroughly wet. The child must be helped to wake and get out of bed as soon as the bell rings (White, 1971). Daily rehearsals can assist the child acquire the habit of getting right up. There should never be more than a small patch of wetness (smaller than a saucer) on the pad. If the wet spot is the size of a dinner plate then the child is not rising quick enough. The child must learn to wake up *quickly* and *completely* to the sound of the bell (Smith, 1974). Make a game out of it and teach the child to "pounce like a cat" on the bell at the first sound.

Experience shows that this problem often improves during treatment since children become more easily alerted as the conditioning proceeds. It is also essential to have an alarm with a very wide range of stimulus intensities. An afternoon nap may be needed if the bed wetter is a deep sleeper.

If the child does not awaken to the alarm, you might try placing a cold wash cloth over the child's forehead and eyes to fully awake him. This should help most children wake up by themselves in three or four days. If the child still does not awaken after a cold wash cloth has been used, it may be necessary for a doctor to prescribe a medication to lighten sleep during the conditioning period. Only about 5 percent of bedwetters will need medication of this kind.

3. Infrequent or Light Wetting. It is very hard to condition a child who wets only two or three times a week, or who is a dribbler (light wetting at night that fails to activate the buzzer). Increasing fluid intake near bedtime to amounts significantly greater than the child's usual intake may help. A diuretic nightly in conjunction with a high fluid intake may be needed to encourage diuresis.

4. Uncooperative Child. Some children may find this treatment a little strange and frightening at first. However, with adequate preparation, a strong fear reaction by the child to the bell and pad is rather uncommon and rarely persists for more than a few days. With very young children the conditioning is usually postponed until the child is four years old. At this age the child shows better understanding, less fear, and better cooperation.

5. Buzzer Ulcers. Cases of buzzer ulcers, that is, painless ulcers on the buttocks, have been reported when the child does not awaken and the skin remains in contact with the urine and the electrical current. One theory is that the wet pad lowers the electrical resistance of the skin (Borrie and Fenton, 1966). Helping the child to quickly awaken to the bell is one approach to this problem. Certain types of equipment will prevent this difficulty.

6. Technical Difficulties. Mechanical problems with the apparatus are not uncommon. The alarm may not go off because of a faulty connection, weak battery, or because the equipment is not sensitive to small amounts of urine. With high quality equipment and close supervison by an experienced therapist, such problems are easily remedied.

7. Dropout Rate. The bell and pad is reported to have a high rate of clients who discontinue treatment (Young and Morgan, 1972; 1973). Azrin and Thienes (1978) state this is because of the long time needed to eliminate enuresis (2 to 3 months), the annoyance caused by parents being awakened in the middle of the night by the alarm, and the inevitable breakdown of the apparatus on occasion. Azrin and Thienes (1978) assert their new rapid method overcomes these difficulties.

8. Treatment not Effective. The bell and pad has not been found to be 100 percent successful and, thus, will not help some children. If after 3 to 4 months there is no sign of improvement, the conditioning should probably be stopped and a complete medical examination be conducted for the possibility of a urinary difficulty.

RETENTION CONTROL TRAINING

There has been some support of late for the 19th century notion of bedwetting as a result of decreased bladder capacity (Glicklich, 1951). Behavioral evidence indicates that some enuretics tend to urinate frequently during the day (Muellner, 1960), while cystometrographic records of bladder pressure and detrusor activity reveal low bladder capacity, with a strong urge to urinate at low bladder pressures and volumes (Stalker and Rand, 1946; Bloomfield and Douglas, 1956). Muellner (1960) states that the tendency to void at low bladder volumes is the primary cause of enuresis. In light of the above, it is reasonable to conclude that if these children are encouraged to retain their urine for longer intervals during the day, this tolerance may carry over to their sleeping state.

Muellner (1960) investigated 327 children ranging in age from two to seven years. He found that when they are able to retain 10 to 12 ounces of urine during the day they are not enuretic at night. He thus recommends that children be given extra fluids during the day and be advised to hold their urine as long as possible so as to promote bladder expansion. With this procedure he reports that these children achieve satisfactory bladder capacity within three to six months. Muellner (1960) monitored bladder capacity by instructing the child to urinate into a measuring cup to demonstrate that he or she was actually voiding larger and larger quantities of urine.

Kimmel and Kimmel (1970) describe a similar but more systematic method of retention control training used in conjunction with reinforcement procedures. They gradually train a child to increase the time between the awareness of the urge to void and the actual micturition. The child is instructed to inform the parent each time it is necessary to empty the bladder during the day. A baseline record of this voiding is kept for at least two days. During the baseline and training periods an unrestricted supply of fluids is made available. The first day of training the child is asked to "Hold it in" for five minutes when told of the urge to urinate. When this is done the child is given a concrete reward selected in advance by the parents, such as cookies, candy, soda. The retention interval is gradually increased in small steps as the child develops the ability to hold more and more urine. The time can be increased in most cases to as much as 30 minutes with a few days training. The size of the reward may also increase. This treatment first results in a decrease in the frequency of daytime urination and then in bedwetting. Success is often achieved within two weeks of training.

Paschalis, Kimmel, and Kimmel (1972) replicated the above study with an additional 31 enuretic children. The retention control training continued until a 45 minute prolongation was attained. The training lasted 20 days and the children were followed up three months later. At this time 15 showed no signs of enuresis and even more showed significant improvement. The training had been administered by the parent with only two hours of instruction by the experimenter. The procedure in this study was as follows. The child determined his or her own initial period of withholding urine. This retention interval was increased by two to three minutes daily until the child could hold for 45 minutes. Tokens and praise were used to reinforce each child immediately at the end of the retention period and just before urination. The tokens were gummed pieces of multicolored paper cut into various sizes, which could be stuck on the pages of an exercise book. At the end of each day the tokens were exchanged for a choice of trinkets. The child recorded his or her withholding time with a marking pen which was kept after charting. The pens were available in a variety of colors, a different color being used each day. At the end of a week of dry nights the child received a gift which had been chosen at the beginning of the training period.

The basic assumption of retention training is that bladder distension constitutes a stimulus for urination and that nocturnal enuretics tend to urinate under conditions of only slight distension. Treatment involves a daytime shaping procedure in which bladder distension cues sufficiently strong to evoke urination are present, but urination is voluntarily withheld. Increasing daytime retention of urine is reinforced on a small step basis, and elimination of nocturnal enuresis tends to follow in a relatively short time.

Stedman (1972) modified the Kimmel and Kimmel procedure for use with older children and adolescents. All monitoring responsibility was given to the 13-year-old girl who had been enuretic all her life. The girl kept a daily diary consisting of a record of bladder distension cues (at three levels—weak, middle, and strong), her frequency of urination, and the number of "accidents" during that week. The first week's record revealed a tendency to urinate frequently and to very weak bladder cues during her waking hours. The girl was then instructed to record distension cues hourly and to discriminate between weak, middle and strong cues. In addition, she was to attempt to retain urine for a 30-minute period beyond the onset of strong bladder distension cues. No control of liquids was made and no tangible reinforcers were given. By the fifth session, daytime frequency of urination had decreased from five to three a day, spaced evenly through the day, and in association with strong bladder cues. Nocturnal enuresis began to decrease rapidly after daytime urination became regular at three a day. No bedwetting occurred after 12 weeks of treatment. A three-month follow-up revealed that the girl had only wet the bed four times during that period.

Miller (1973) found that retention control training resulted in marked decreases in both daytime urinations and bedwetting episodes in two institutionalized adolescents. After 11 weeks of treatment the enuresis disappeared in both cases and this success was still apparent at a seven-month follow-up.

In Miller's study, the subjects recorded the incidence of bedwetting each night and the frequency of daytime urinations. The subjects were instructed to "hold back" urination for 10 minutes each time they felt an urge to urinate during the daytime. After the waiting period they were to go to the bathroom as usual. During the second and third weeks of treatment this time interval was increased to 20 and 30 minutes, respectively. The children were also instructed to increase their consumptions of fluids (cokes, water, etc.) during the day. It was assumed that increased fluid intake would lead to more urges to urinate and therefore more learning trials. The therapist praised and encouraged the subjects for their efforts at "holding back" for the specified time periods. Treatment was discontinued after three consecutive weeks of no bed wetting.

Doleys and Wells (1975) asked the parents of a three-year-old girl to measure the magnitude of each voiding incident before, during and after retention control training. The mean amount per occurrence increased from about 1.5 ounces (44 ml) during baseline to nearly 4 ounces (118 ml) for the last four days of a 21-day period of retention control training combined with forced liquids. The average child this age can retain 3.5 ounces of urine. Dry nights were not associated with increased bladder capacity and occurred only after the parents began to awaken the child and place her on the toilet twice a night. Once achieved, however, nocturnal continence was maintained when awakening and toileting were terminated. The magnitude of nighttime urinations was found below post-training daytime mean but well above the pretraining daytime mean.

In addition to retaining urine for long intervals, some therapists recommend strengthening the sphincter muscle of the bladder by having the child practice starting and stopping the flow of urine. For example, Chapman (1974) suggests showing the child a sketch

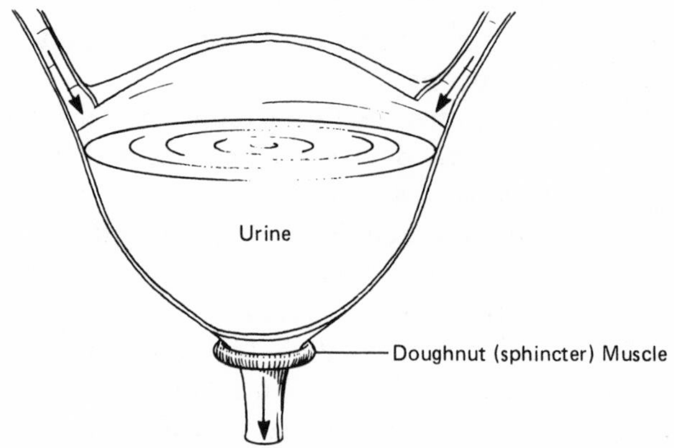

Figure 5. Sketch of the Bladder.

of the bladder (Figure 5), and explaining that the urine comes out when the doughnut (sphincter) muscle opens up. The child is told that the bedwetting is not his fault but, rather, is due to a weak doughnut muscle. It needs to be strengthened by exercise to make it strong. The child is told to practice stopping micturition in midstream and starting it, then stopping again. The child is to do this stop-start routine over and over during daytime micturition, and it is suggested that this will strengthen the bladder muscle and that bedwetting will stop. Chapman suggests allowing several months for this to work.

In conclusion, while the retention or bladder stretching procedure does seem promising, there is need for further investigation of its general applicability. The approach needs careful recording and close supervision to be effective. Also, some parents may find it hard to ask their child to hold urine "until it hurts" or is uncomfortable.

DRUG TREATMENT

As long as there have been enuretic children there have been drug treatments offered to them. Today, however, drugs have a rather undistinguished record in the treatment of nocturnal enuresis (Meadow, 1974). The tricyclic antidepressants are the only drugs that have been consistently shown to be superior to placebo (Blackwell and Curragh, 1973). Imipramine (Tofranil) is the most commonly used. Although Imipramine tends to reduce the number of wet nights in many children, total dryness is less frequent. Also, many children relapse and resume wetting once the drug is discontinued (Alderton, 1965). Forsythe and Redmond (1974) report that some 10 to 40 percent of the children treated with this drug have greater than a 50 percent reduction in bedwetting, but they tend to relapse when treatment is withdrawn. Olness (1975) cautioned against the use of Imipramine because of the temporary effect, the fact that the FDA has not approved this drug for children under 12, and in light of the findings that it has caused numerous deaths when accidentally ingested by toddlers and unstable older children in the home.

Imipramine is an anticholinergic drug, and its mode of action is not presently known (Shaffer, 1970). There is some evidence that it effects the reticular and hypothalamic systems, the latter, according to Agarwala and Heycock (1968), having "marked control over micturition (p. 296)." In regard to physical effects, anticholinergic drugs relax the detrusor muscle of the urinary bladder and increase the tonicity of the internal sphincter of the bladder. This combined effect permits the bladder to hold a greater quantity of urine before the "stretch reflex" induces the bladder to contract and urination occurs (Agarwala and Heycock, 1968). Others (Tec, 1964) report that it decreases the depth of sleep and so assists in the effort to maintain sphincter control.

According to Meadow (1974), a simple drug treatment is to use a starting dose of 25 mg. Imipramine. The dose is increased at fortnightly intervals by 25 mg. up to a maximum dose of 75 mg. The most common reason for having to stop the drug is the onset of mood or sleep disturbance as the dose is increased. If the child regularly wets before midnight it may be better to give the drug at 4:00 p.m. Alderton (1967) found that by dividing enuretic children into two groups according to the time at which they characteristically wet the bed (early or late) and administering the drug about 5 hours before that time, he could obtain his best results. Among the side effects of Tofranil are reduced appetite, weight loss, sleeplessness, irritability and skin rashes.

Next to antidepressants, the stimulants are the most widely used drugs. The three major reasons for their use are: (1) to lighten sleep so as to permit easier waking; (2) to stimulate sphincter control, and; (3) to quicken the acquisition of a conditioned response in bell and pad conditioning. Pierce *et al.* (1961) used amphetamines to lighten sleep intensity in the belief that the impulse from a full bladder would wake the light sleeping child. Young and Turner (1965) found that central nervous system stimulant drugs facilitate the conditioning process when the urine alarm is used. Methedrine was found to be slightly superior to Dexedrine.

Although stimulant drugs may be successful initially, the child usually develops tolerance to the drug so that larger and larger doses are necessary to achieve the desired result. The effect of amphetamines is often short-lived, and enuresis usually recurs as soon as the medication is stopped. These drugs also cause irritability and restlessness and make it difficult for the child to get a sufficient amount of sleep at night, resulting in irritability and lethargy the next day.

In summary, a wide variety of drugs have been used in the treatment of enuresis. However, only the tricyclic antidepressants have been found to be superior to placebo in the treatment of enuresis (Blackwell, 1971; Brown and Ford-Smith, 1941). Unfortunately, the effects of the antidepressants tend to be suppressive rather than curative and, once the medication is stopped, relapse is the rule rather than the exception (Forsythe and Merrett, 1969). Nevertheless, drugs can play a role in treating enuresis. For example, they can be helpful with children who need to be dry for a particular occasion such as a camp, for those who are unable to use the bell and pad because of the home situation, or to lighten sleep and facilitate conditioning.

PSYCHODYNAMIC APPROACH

The aim of the psychodynamically oriented therapist is to identify psychological disturbances at the root of the enuresis. A basic premise is that bedwetting is an overt sign of some underlying conflict or emotional problem, such as unconscious passive-aggressive reactions toward parents, castration fears related to an oedipal conflict (English and Pearson, 1945), or regressive reactions to threat (Gerard, 1959).

Some dynamically oriented therapists have attempted to discredit conditioning procedures with enuresis on the grounds that enuresis is a symptom of a deeper, internal problem. Thus, by removing only the symptom, the cause will remain and emerge in the form of a different symptom. Studies, however, have consistently failed to reveal any evidence of symptom substitution (Doleys, 1977). On the contrary, children relieved of enuresis have been found to become happier, less anxious, more responsible and adventuresome, and more self-confident (Baker, 1969).

Studies comparing the effectiveness of psychotherapy and the bell and pad procedure have consistently favored the latter. For instance, Werry and Cohrssen (1965) compared the bell and pad procedure with supportive psychotherapy. Psychotherapy consisted of six to eight sessions of psychodynamically oriented therapy supplemented with suggestion and encouragement over a three-month interval. The no-treatment and psychotherapy groups were statistically indistinguishable in regard to the elimination of bedwetting, while the bed and pad procedure was found to be superior to both of these groups.

Most enuretic children show little sign of psychopathology, so that prolonged, expensive dynamically oriented treatment seems both unnecessary and undesirable. There is generally no need to make children undergo what is often an unpleasant social and personal experience for them and a highly expensive experience for their parents (Werry, 1967). Only if severe psychological problems are present in addition to the enuresis does psychoanalytic or family therapy seem warranted.

CONTINGENCY MANAGEMENT

If the child does not wet every night and keeping dry seems within his or her ability, some therapists recommend using contingency management procedures (Ross, 1974). Contingency management involves giving the child rewards for dry nights and/or penalties for wet nights.

Rewards

Popler (1976) gave token rewards for nonenuretic behavior to a 14-year-old male with a lifelong history of bedwetting. Initially the child recorded the incidence of wet and dry nights over a two-month baseline period. Once treatment was begun the boy continued to maintain his own records and to visit the therapist once a week. He received one coupon from the therapist for each dry night that week. After collecting 15 coupons he could turn them in for $5.00 cash. The coupon requirement was then raised to 20 and then 35. The boy and his parents were reinterviewed every two months to discuss his progress. A chart of his progress was maintained by the boy in the therapist's office. During treatment the number of dry nights gradually increased until they averaged six or seven by week thirteen. After week 23 the tokens were eliminated but the parents were advised to continue verbal praise for dry nights. From week 24 on, the boy was completely dry at night and therapy sessions were terminated at week 28. The boy was still dry at a six month follow-up and seemed more confident, had more friends, and was doing better in school.

Bach and Moylan (1975) used contingent rewards to eliminate bedwetting behavior in a six-year-old boy who was also encopretic. After a discussion of the principles of operant conditioning with the parents, the agreed upon reinforcer was money. The therapists explained to the boy he would receive a quarter for ever BM in the toilet, 10¢ for every urination in the commode, and 10¢ for every morning his bed was not wet. The parents gave these reinforcers directly after the behavior occurred and praised the child. All inappropriate eliminations were ignored by the parents and the boy's clothes were changed as perfunctorily as possible. This program was carried out for 12 weeks and was successful in bringing the bedwetting under control. After some minor changes in the monetary rewards, the encopresis was also brought under control by this method. The parents were reported to feel a tremendous sense of accomplishment after three years of frustration in attempting to reduce the boy's elimination difficulties.

Other therapists recommend that parents reward a child for dry nights by the use of social reinforcers, such as praise and attention. The use of social reinforcers to night train a child is, of course, not new. Indeed, Benjamin, Serdahely, and Geppert (1971) found that the most effective reinforcers used by normal parents to night train children are hugging, kissing and praising the child when successful at achieving a dry night. It was noted that negative reinforcers such as shaming, rejecting, spanking, and name calling, significantly retarded night training. Restricting fluids after dinner, waking the child before the parents retired, or stopping the night bottle did not seem to help the training. It was discovered that having a motivated child, that is, one eager to be dry and concerned about accidents, and making the child responsible for his/her own training ("It is up to the child to train self"), were positively related to success. Typically, the parents began night training when the child was two years old and training was usually completed after 3 to 4 months. A discriminative stimulus such as switching the child from diapers to training pants at night was also related to success. The authors of this study conclude that the operant conditioning model is implicitly present in the way most children are toilet trained, and the most effective reinforcers are those which are interpersonal in nature.

Penalties

Allgeier (1976) used a behavior modification procedure for enuresis which consisted of a penalty or response cost contingency for bedwetting. A 20-week period was needed to treat two sisters, 8 and 11 years old. Each morning for the first five weeks the girls indicated whether or not they had wet the bed by signing a chart on the refrigerator. They were penalized 10¢ (one-tenth of their allowance) if they did not sign in and 50¢ if they did not tell the truth, which was determined by having the parents periodically check the bedding. The parents strictly enforced the morning recording but did not comment on the presence or absence of bedwetting.

After the initial five weeks when the signing in had been firmly established, another penalty was imposed. The girls were not allowed any liquid intake after 6:00 p.m. (bedtime was 9:00 p.m.) until they had been continent for 21 consecutive nights. The parents enforced this contingency and the daily sign-ins. The girls were able to monitor their own behavior accurately and consistently, and they became quite interested in the process. Results showed the 11-year-old exhibited a steady decline in wetting through the first five weeks, from five incidences a week to two. After two episodes during the first week of no evening liquids, she remained dry except for one accident during the 11th week. The eight-year-old followed the same pattern but was a bit more variable. At the termination of the program the eight-year-old had been dry for 44 nights and her sister had been dry for 65 nights. The author states that the main advantage of this method is that it minimizes the time required by adults to supervise the training.

In regard to the use of penalties or unpleasant consequences following bedwetting, it should be noted that many therapists consider the bell and pad procedure to be an operant approach whereby aversive consequences are applied *immediately* after bedwetting occurs.

NIGHTLY AWAKENING

Some parents develop the habit of "lifting" their bedwetting child at night, that is, taking the child to the toilet to urinate without waking the child. The effect of this practice according to White (1971), is to train the child to urinate while asleep. In White's study, a total of 287 of the 1,000 mothers interviewed admitted using this practice with children over five years old. Other adults will wake the child to void at a fixed time each night.

Simply awakening children at a certain time each night, say two hours after bedtime, is also ineffective in eliminating bedwetting.

Although the awakening tends to reduce the frequency of wetting at night, there is usually a rapid increase in bedwetting once the procedure is halted.

Young (1964) developed a staggered-wakening technique whereby the enuretic child is awakened each night for four weeks at different times to get the child used to waking up with different bladder pressures. Initially the children were awakened three times per night but the number of awakenings was gradually reduced until they were not awakened at all at the end of treatment. The results showed that 67 percent of the 58 enuretic children treated improved, with 10 children being completely dry after two or three nights of the treatment.

Creer and Davis (1975) replicated the method with enuretic children in an institutional setting. Previous efforts to treat the problem by the use of drugs or awakening the children once each night at a fixed time had proven unsuccessful. Initially, the children were awakened three times each night, according to a variable interval schedule. The exact times were selected by drawing numbers from a hat. After two weeks, a fading procedure was initiated, whereby the children were awakened only twice a night. The third stage, begun two weeks later, involved awakening the children only once each night for a period of two weeks. The final one-month period consisted of allowing the children to sleep undisturbed at night.

The results of this study disclosed that the staggered wakening approach produced a significant decrease in bedwetting both during the treatment period and over the one-month follow up. Most of the children maintained their gains when they returned home. Creer and Davis hypothesize that the method was effective because the children found it quite aversive to be awakened on a frequent and unpredictable basis. McConaghy (1969), however, reports that a similar random wakening procedure was effective with only one of five children, and that the bell and pad method was much superior.

Rather than staggering nightly wakenings some therapists suggest checking on a child at regular intervals during the night, and waking the child up if the bed is wet. Like the bell and pad procedure, it is hoped that the child will find such awakenings aversive and stop wetting the bed.

Catalina (1976) for example, used the following parent administered waking procedure. For a two-week baseline recording period the parents made three nighttime observations. The first observation of wetting was made two to three hours after bedtime, 11 to 12 p.m.; the second at 3 to 4 a.m.; the third at 6 to 7 a.m., preferably before the child awoke. Without the child's knowledge, the parents recorded date and time of observation, occurrence and estimated size of wet spot; a sleep level code, and relevant notes. The therapist then met with the child and parents and explained the basal observation process and its purpose to the child. The parents continued the nightly observations for at least two more weeks. They did not awaken the child.

At this point the therapist met with the parents and child and explained the training procedure. The parents were to continue the three nightly observations; now, however, when the child was found wet he/she was to be awakened, informed of being wet, sent to the bathroom, and assisted in remaking the bed upon return. The cooperative and helping aspects of the procedure were stressed. The therapist suggested changes in the time of the second observation to minimize delay between wetting and awakening. Results showed seven of 20 children (35 percent) stopped wetting after an average training of 134 days. Eleven children (55 percent) did not become dry after at least 13 weeks of training. Two children were still training at 25 and 28 weeks. The results indicated that the success rate was below most bell and pad studies and training took longer. The fact that awakening was not immediate after wetting in this study would seem to account for the poorer performance as compared with the bell and pad. Also, the machine can detect more wettings and, thus, produce more conditioning experiences.

Samaan (1972), however, reports the case of a seven-year-old enuretic girl for whom previous psychoanalytic, bell and pad, and drug treatment had been unsuccessful in reducing the enuresis. Since the child liked chocolate more than anything else to eat, and liked body touch, a contingency procedure was set up. After one hour of going to bed the child was awakened by the parents and guided between their arms to the bathroom. As she started urinating, a piece of chocolate was given her. The gentle awakening and walk to the bathroom for reinforced urination were repeated every night at two to three-hour intervals. A gentle hug was given after awakening. On the fourth day the chocolate was put on the water tank and the child was directed to take it herself. After 10 days the parents waited to see if the child woke up spontaneously after one hour. If not, they followed the usual procedure. During the second week the parents woke the child three times intermittently, and in the fourth week, the child started to get up on her own to go to the bathroom while the parents intermittently praised her. Every morning they hugged and praised her to show their pleasure. From the fifth through the seventh week, candy was given only occasionally. By the eighth week the candy was only given the child in the morning coupled with praise. After three accidents during the first three weeks when the parents failed to follow the requirements, the child remained dry, and this continued during the two-year follow-up. The parents continued the procedure for a year to ensure the child was confidently in contol of her urination.

Some therapists use a nighttime wake-up procedure to train a child to retain urine at night for longer and longer intervals. The goal is similar to the retention control training described earlier, only the problem of generalization from daytime to nighttime control is avoided. For instance, Singh, Phillips, and Fischer (1976) switched from Kimmel's daytime retention training procedure to a nocturnal wake-up procedure and obtained good results with the latter. Since the girl, age 13, regularly wet two to three hours after retiring, she was instructed to set her alarm to go off two hours after bedtime. She was to go to the toilet when the alarm rang and then return to sleep until morning (approximately 6:00 a.m.). After seven consecutive dry nights, she was to set the alarm at 90 minutes after bedtime. Seven consecutive dry nights were the criterion for each further reduction in time to 60 minutes after bedtime, 45 minutes and, finally, 30 minutes. She was then to go to the toilet without the alarm clock every other night in an effort to fade out its use.

The girl did not wet for seven nights when the alarm was set for two hours. She wet three times when it was set for 90 minutes. At 60 minutes, after one wetting incident the first week, she completed seven consecutive dry nights. At 45 minutes there was also one wetting incident the first week only. At 30 minutes she had no accidents. At this point she agreed to clean the bedsheets and was promised a new bed by her parents for six months of no wetting. Her parents praised her for dry nights and the therapist did similarly when he called once a week. After one week of dry nights the alarm clock use was faded. During the next two months she did not wet.

An eight-month follow-up revealed no relapse. Due to several interruptions for vacations, the treatment period spanned 15 months.

In conclusion, of all the wake-up procedures, the ones which directly teach the retention of urine at night seem most promising.

COUNSELING APPROACH

The counseling approach to treating enuresis has four main goals. The first is to *provide support* to parents and child by such means as giving encouragement, relieving guilt and developing a positive expectancy of success. The second goal is to *give information* about such topics as effective toilet training practices, causes of enuresis and physiology of the bladder. The third objective is to *promote independence* by having the parents administer the treatment and giving the child as much responsibility as possible for his or her own treatment. The final goal is to *develop rapport* with the parent and child which is characterized by mutual respect, trust and liking. You show the family that you are deeply interested in them as persons and that you are a person worthy of being identified with.

Supportive therapy has been successfully combined with bell and pad conditioning to treat persistent enuretics (Novick, 1966). The conditioning procedure was employed only when necessary. The supportive therapy was aimed at relieving the child's guilt, increasing his self-confidence, and at becoming the child's ally by dissuading the parents from using punitive and harsh toilet training procedures. Only four of 45 children so treated failed to reach a cure criterion of 14 consecutive dry nights. Primary enuretic children required twice as long (mean of 46 days) to reach the criterion as did the secondary enuretics (mean of 23 days).

Dische (1971) used advice and encouragement which involved instructing the parents to be matter-of-fact about wetting episodes and not to punish the wetter. The child charted his wetting and had regular contact with the therapist, during which he was reinforced for dry nights. Thirty-seven percent of the children treated were dried up in this manner, with only one child showing a relapse. The remaining 79 children were treated with the urine alarm and 92 percent were successfully treated. Other studies have also reported success with encouragement-type therapy (Meadow, 1970; White, 1971). But the procedure is not clearly defined and rather low success rates are often reported. However it does seem to be a fact that some children can be helped by encouragement therapy, thus making it potentially useful in practice. It should be recognized that failure with this form of treatment may adversely effect later therapeutic interventions.

Advice Giving

In regard to advice giving, some families may not know the following:

1. The use of harsh punishment, shaming or ridicule when a child wets can exacerbate the problem.

2. Restricting fluids at bedtime is not helpful. Indeed, Hagglund (1965) showed that fluid restriction may exacerbate the enuresis problem by inducing bladder neck irritation and the urge to micturate at lower than normal volumes of bladder urine.

Positive reinforcement for dry nights seems much more effective in the long run.

3. The child is not wetting the bed because he is lazy or obstinate or rebellious. It is most likely because his bladder control is slow in developing and has become anxious about the problem. The child should be clearly told that the problem is not his fault.

The family should understand that enuresis is a very common childhood problem and, that, typically, it is not a sign of an underlying emotional disturbance.

4. There are a number of very effective treatment methods for enuresis and the odds are very high that the problem can be corrected within a few months.

5. Facts about the basic physiology of the bladder can help one understand the problem.

Responsibility Training

Dimson (1959) showed that enuretic children differed from a control group not by virtue of the age at which toilet training was commenced or the severity with which it was administered, but rather in the amount of resistance the children had put up to the process. So it seems very important for successful toilet training that the child have an inner motivation to be dry and a sense of personal responsibility for achieving this dryness. While Dollard and Miller (1950) have described the theoretical rationale of this inner motivation, others have attempted to incorporate it as part of the treatment for enuresis.

Marshall, Marshall and Lyon (1973), for example, developed an approach termed responsibility-reinforcement. The overall goal is to make the child an active vs. passive participant in therapy. This method combines principles derived from two schools of thought: (1) reality therapy principles which emphasize the child's assuming responsibility for his own behavior; and (2) techniques of positive reinforcement and response shaping from behavior modification theory.

If the child seems eager to change his bedwetting habits and wants to take responsibility himself, the first step is for the child to maintain a progress record. When he does record a wet night on the chart, he is to try to determine the causes leading to this, such as a stressful day. When he is dry the child affixes a star on the chart or calendar. The discussions and encouragement of the therapist serve to reinforce the successes achieved. In addition, a response-shaping procedure is used, that is, a step-by-step change in behavior toward a given goal by means of rewards for each successive level of improvement. To lengthen sleep intervals while dry, an alarm clock is set so the child awakens and empties his bladder at longer and longer intervals. These increasing intervals are recorded by the child on the chart. Recording this progressive improvement is a reward in itself, but the family and therapist also reinforce the progress.

An additional technique of assuming responsibility for treatment is "sensation awareness." To encourage the child to be more aware of the sensation of a full bladder, he is encouraged to hold his urine as long as possible during the day, and then void into a measuring cup and record the maximum volume. Whether or not an actual increase in bladder capacity is achieved, this method has the effect of making the child acutely aware of the sensation of bladder distension. Furthermore, by stopping and starting his stream at will during micturition, the child can become more conscious of his power to control the act of voiding.

The authors considered a child to have shown marked improvement if there was a monthly decrease of enuresis of more than 80 percent; an improvement if there was a 40 to 80 percent decrease, and a failure if less than a 40 percent decrease was evident. They found that responsibility-reinforcement therapy resulted in slightly better success rates than more passive forms such as the bell and pad. The training took longer but it resulted in a lower relapse rate (about 5 percent) than the other forms of treatment.

When a child takes an active responsibility for seeking to change his behavior and is supported by positive reinforcement from parents and therapist, there seems to be more positive benefits to his self-esteem and self-development than if he is a passive participant in the therapy, as with conditioning and drug treatment. Improvement in the latter groups is frequently more rapid but the relapse rate seems to be higher than in the responsibility-reinforcement approach. The latter seems less disruptive from a psychological as well as physiological point of view. However, in the responsibility-reinforcement approach, the child must want to stop bedwetting and take responsibility for it happening.

HYPNOSIS

Hypnosis has been reported as a highly successful treatment for enuresis (Collins, 1970; Kroger, 1963). Olness (1975) used a self-hypnosis technique with 40 enuretic children, ages 4½ to 16 years. The two teenagers in the group were taught a standard hand levitation technique to induce self-hypnosis. The coin technique was used with the 38 younger children. Olness (1975) describes the coin procedure as follows (pp. 274–275):

> "The child was seated in a comfortable chair alongside the physician who was also seated. With a marking pencil, a "clown face" was drawn on his right or left thumbnail (depending on his preference). A quarter was then placed between his thumb and forefinger, and he was asked to hold the quarter up in front of his face in such a way that he was looking at the face on the thumbnail. He was told that he was to focus only on the face and that, as he did so, the quarter would slowly become heavy and would slip down and fall. When this happened he would feel very relaxed and his eyes would close. As he looked at the picture on the thumbnail, he was encouraged by saying that he had an excellent attention span, that he was becoming very relaxed, and that the quarter was getting heavier and heavier. He was told not to worry if the quarter fell on the floor and that when he became relaxed

and closed his eyes he should put his hands on his thighs. He would then be asked questions which he could answer by raising his yes hand or his no hand. This was done in order to acquaint the child with the hand raising technique. When the quarter fell, which usually occurred within five minutes, a number of questions were asked, most of which were non sequiturs: "Do you like the color yellow?", "Do you like to eat ice cream?", "Do you like to eat salad?", "Do you like to go to bed?", and, finally, "Would you like to have dry beds every night?" If the answer was affirmative, he was told, "You have learned this trick very quickly, and you can use it to have dry beds every night. The reason you sometimes have wet beds is that you do not wake up at night when you need to urinate (or equivalent word which the child would understand). I would like you to do this trick every night before you go to bed and tell yourself the following things when the quarter falls down: 'When I need to urinate I will wake up all by myself, go to the bathroom all by myself, urinate in the toilet, and return to my nice dry bed. I will go back to sleep. If I need to urinate another time, I will wake up all by myself, urinate in the toilet, and return to my dry bed. When I wake up, my bed will be dry and I will be very happy.' After you have finished telling yourself these things, imagine the feeling you have when you wake up and your bed is dry. It's a comfortable good feeling. When you finish your imagining, open your eyes."

Olness (1975) asked the child to do the above procedure every night until the next appointment. The parents were asked not to remind the child, because it was up to him whether or not he wished to use this trick. The parents were also advised not to comment on the condition of the bed (wet or dry) unless the child raised the issue. Follow-up office visits were made every one to two weeks until the beds were dry (defined as no more than one wet bed per month), and then monthly for as long as the child desired. During each visit the child was asked how many dry beds he had since the last appointment. At these follow-up visits the technique of self-hypnosis or self-conditioning was reviewed and the children were praised for success. The visits only lasted five to ten minutes. The results indicated that 31 of the 40 children were cured of bedwetting, six showed substantial improvement, and three did not improve. Of the

31 who completely ceased bedwetting, 28 did so in the first month of treatment. Thirty-six of the 38 children who learned the coin technique became very proficient at achieving self-relaxation after one or two visits and could drop the coin in less than two minutes. Most of the children exhibited new confidence at having achieved the cure on their own.

Olness (1977) reports a 90 percent success rate with this method in treating over 200 enuretic children. She states that clinicians interested in the method need to study basic hypnosis theory and practice in workshops sponsored by such groups as the American Society of Clinical Hypnosis or the Society of Clinical and Experimental Hypnosis.

It should also be noted that hypnotism is sometimes combined with other techniques. Schwidder (1953) employed hypnoanalysis successfully in the treatment of a 16-year-old male enuretic. Only one 90-minute session was required to stop bedwetting, but psychoanalytic therapy was continued for some sessions to ensure against relapse. The focus of the analysis was on the adolescent's repressed wishes for love and security and on his tendency to submit to aggression with a passive-dependent reaction.

COMBINED APPROACHES

In most bell and pad studies the urine alarm was the only form of intervention employed, although James and Foreman (1973) report that therapist variables are associated with different outcomes in the use of this apparatus. In recent years, therapists have been experimenting with the use of adjunct methods. Browning (1967), for example, tried a reinforcement system in which the child, who previously did not awaken to the bell, was reinforced with points for responding to the alarm and given extra points for each dry night. Accumulated points were then exchangeable for items on a reinforcement menu. Kimmel and Kimmel (1970) administered a variety of rewards to motivate children to endure their retention control training. Supportive therapy has been successfully combined with bell and pad conditioning to treat persistent enuretics (Novick, 1966). Other therapists use drugs in combination with the urine alarm.

Crandall (1946) obtained an 80 percent cure rate using a combination of dietary, conditioning, suggestion, and medical approaches.

He restricted fluid intake after evening meals, prohibited the eating of raw apples, canned fish, candy, ice cream, pepper and other condiments, and the drinking of coffee, tea, cocoa, and cola drinks. The children were instructed to eat a light supper, but were free to eat salty foods such as popcorn before bedtime. Regular daily "toilet-times" were set for each child and all were to urinate just prior to bedtime each night. During the day the children were instructed to pinch themselves several times whenever they felt the urge to urinate. Upon going to bed for the night, each child was instructed to repeat to himself several times: "I'm going to wake up at (some preselected time during the night)." No rough play was allowed after supper. Efforts were made to correct any physical disorders and to bring weight up to normal. Vitamins were given daily, especially A, B complex and D. Cold sleeping quarters and heavy bedclothes were avoided and each boy was required to launder his own bed linens and soiled clothing himself.

To speed up the effectiveness of the urine alarm apparatus, Azrin, Sneed and Foxx, (1974) added several other procedures such as training in inhibiting urination, positive reinforcement for correct urination, training in rapid awakening, increased fluid intake, increased social motivation to be nonenuretic, self-correction of accidents, and practice in toileting. A study showed that after one all-night training session, the 24 enuretic children averaged only two bedwettings before achieving 14 consecutive dry nights. This intensive procedure called dry-bed training, was found to be a more rapid and effective treatment as compared with the use of the bell and pad alone. Azrin and his associates have found it particularly effective with mentally retarded populations and Butler (1976b) used Azrin's procedure to toilet train a child with Spina Bifida.

Bollard and Woodroffe (1977) modified the dry bed training in that they had parents administer the intense all-night training program rather than an outside trainer. With 14 children treated in this manner, the bedwetting was eliminated in all cases—within an average of 12 days. There were two relapses after six months. They also investigated the effect of eliminating the adjunct bell and pad machine from the dry-bed training. This resulted in a significant reduction in the frequency of bedwetting, although the bed wetting was not completely eliminated in any of the 10 children treated. So parent-administered dry-bed training shows promise of being a more efficient and effective treatment of nocturnal enuresis than alternate methods, including the standard bell and pad method, drug treatment and psychotherapy (Bollard and Woodroffe, 1977).

The Azrin procedure is complex in that it uses a variety of different procedures. Thus, it is difficult to assess which aspect, if any, contributes most heavily to the success of treatment. If it can be assumed that children will respond differently to each technique, then dry-bed training may be uniquely capable of being effective with a wide range of children.

Doleys, Ciminero, Tollison, Williams and Wells (1977) replicated the dry-bed training procedure using 13 children. There was a substantial decrease in wetting after six weeks of treatment, but the results were not as remarkable as those reported by Azrin *et al.* (1974). The authors report a substantially longer time to treat and a lower rate of success than did Azrin, indicating the need for further investigation.

Recently, Azrin and Thienes (1978) modified the dry-bed training to make it more convenient to use by eliminating the bell and pad conditioning. The new method consists of one day of intensive training, and involves a combination of reinforcement for inhibiting urination, practice in appropriate urination, bladder awareness training, copious drinking, self-correction and positive practice for accidents, awakening training, and family encouragement. The steps in the new procedure are presented in Table 3. Azrin and Thienes report that this method quickly and consistently eliminates enuresis in children who are age three or over. The average child has only four bedwetting incidents before achieving two weeks of dryness. Relapses are infrequent (20 percent) and always reversed by a second training session.

Table 3. New Treatment Steps.
(Adopted from Azrin and Thienes, 1978)

I. Training day
   A. Afternoon
      1. Parents and child are informed of the entire procedure
      2. Child is encouraged to drink favorite beverage to increase urination
      3. Child is requested to attempt initiation of urination every .5 hour
         a) If child feels the need to urinate, he is asked to hold for increasingly longer periods of time
         b) If child has to urinate, he is asked to lie in bed as if he were asleep then jump up and go to the bathroom, role-playing what he should do at night. He then is rewarded with a beverage and praise

Table 3. (Cont'd)

4. Child is motivated to work at dry beds
   a) Parents and child review inconveniences caused by bedwetting
   b) Parents contract with the child for rewards to be given after first dry night and after a specified series of dry nights
   c) Child specifies persons he'd like to tell when he can keep dry
   d) Child is given a chart to mark to show his progress posting this in a prominent spot.

B. One hour before bedtime with parents watching
1. Child is informed of all phases of maintenance procedures
2. Child role-plays cleanliness training
   a) Child is required to put on own pajamas
   b) Child is required to remove sheets and put them back on
3. Child role-plays positive practice in toileting
   a) Child lies down in bed as if asleep (lights out)
   b) Child counts to 50
   c) Child arises and hurries to bathroom where he attempts urination
   d) Child returns to bed
   e) Steps a-d repeated 20 times with parent counting trials

C. At bedtime
1. Child repeats instructions on accident correction and nighttime awakenings to trainer.
2. Child continues to drink fluids
3. Parents talk to child about rewards and their confidence in child
4. Comments on dryness of sheets
5. Child retires for the night

D. Hourly awakenings 'til 1 a.m.
1. If child is dry
   a) Minimal prompt is used to awaken
   b) Child is asked what he should do
      (1) If can wait another hour
         (a) Trainer praises his urinary control
         (b) Child returns to bed
      (2) If must urinate
         (a) Child goes to bathroom
         (b) Trainer praises him for correct toileting
         (c) Child returns to bed
      (3) Child feels bed sheets and comments on their dryness
      (4) Trainer praises child for having dry bed
      (5) Child is given fluids (after 11 pm discontinue beverages)
      (6) Child returns to sleep
2. When an accident has occurred
   a) Parent awakens child and reprimands him for wetting
   b) Parent directs child to bathroom to finish urinating
   c) Child is given cleanliness training
      (1) Child changes night clothes
      (2) Child removes wet sheets and places them in dirty laundry

Table 3. (Cont'd)

(3) Child obtains clean sheets and remakes bed

d) Positive practice in correct toileting (20 trials) is performed immediately after cleanliness training

e) Child is reminded that positive practice is necessary before bed the following evening

E. Parents check the child .5 hour early the next morning

II. Post-training parental supervision

A. If dry in the morning

1. Point out to child .5 hour before usual bedtime that he may stay up that extra .5 hour because he needn't practice and would be awakened .5 hour earlier that night
2. Point out his chart to show his progress toward rewards
3. Tell visitors to the home how he is keeping his bed dry
4. Bring his success up at least three times a day

B. If wet in the morning

1. Wake him .5 hour early asking him what he should do and to feel his sheets
2. Child is required to change his bed and pajamas
3. Child does positive practice in correct toileting (20 trials)
4. Child does positive practice (20 trials) .5 hour before bed that night
5. Child marks chart and is told we will try again tomorrow
6. Tell visitors to the home that the child is learning to keep his bed dry

Although the dry-bed procedure is quite innovative and promising, a big disadvantage of this training is that it places a considerable drain on the time and energy of parents or staff. Also, Matson and Ollendick (1977) report that certain aspects of Azrin's toilet training procedures, such as 20 positive practice sessions, can be quite adversive to children. Preschool children may react to such methods with temper tantrums, hitting or avoidance behavior. Since Butler (1976) reports that parents may become upset by the procedure as well, close supervision and support by a therapist is needed for the successful application of dry-bed training. While this method seems uniquely effective with certain "hard to train" children, there is a continuing need for a method that requires less effort to implement and monitor. Until such a method is discovered, the bell and pad will probably remain the method of choice for general use in light of its high success rate without adjunct methods.

In conclusion, the use of a variety of techniques in combination with one another may maximize the generality of the treatment method to more varied population and settings. It is still not clear how much, if any, adjunct procedures help the standard bell and pad procedure, but there is some evidence to suggest it can be useful with certain cases.

The clinician skilled in a variety of techniques is in a position to differentially apply treatment methods in various combinations and sequences, in accord with the needs of the individual case (Shepherd and Durham, 1977). Of course, there is a need for assessment procedures that can form the basis for differential application of specific procedures. At the present time it seems that the "hard-to-train" child is best treated by a combination of techniques.

4

Summary and Conclusions

Enuresis and encopresis present a serious threat to the emotional adjustment of a child. Thus, to allow a child to wrestle with the problem for five to ten years while he or she is hopefully to outgrow the habit is, to say the least, a course of action hard to justify. For instance, to recommend to the parents of a five-year-old child with enuresis that they should ignore the problem because he/she will probably outgrow it, gives the child only a 50-50 chance of achieving dryness over the next five years. For some of these children the problem will persist into adulthood. On the other hand, effective treatment approaches now exist which can bring about success within a period of months.

A recent survey (Yankelovich, Skelly, and White, 1977) revealed that most parents do not seek outside advice when their children exhibit behavior problems at home, rather, they attempt to handle it alone. Thus, it is not unusual for a child to suffer with a bedwetting problem through the grade school years. It is obvious that greater use will have to be made of the mass media to bring to the attention of the American family the fact that effective methods are now available to relieve bedwetting difficulties, and to put parents in touch with local sources of professional assistance.

There are a number of experienced and enthusiastic therapists throughout the country who are skilled in a variety of different stratagems and can use them with confidence in accord with the needs of the particular child and family.

Of the different treatments used to date, the bell and pad conditioning method has the most favorable record of success both in terms of the child's initial attainment of dryness and in regard to the stability of the correction. However, as Olness (1977) states, it is naive to think that one treatment will work equally well with all children. Certain children do not respond to the bell and pad method and some parents will not try it. Enuretic children with mental or neurological deficiencies, in particular, seem to respond best to a more intense approach. Thus, the differential application of the many available treatment methods, based upon diagnostic information of the individual case, is starting to be discussed in the literature (Doleys, *et al.*, 1977). Other therapists suggest that it is best to have a continuum of interventions available and to initially use the least disruptive or aversive method.

ASPECTS OF EFFECTIVE TREATMENT

In treating the enuretic child it seems advisable from the available evidence to keep in mind the following points:

1. Conduct an initial interview to assess such factors as the history and previous treatment of enuresis, toilet training practices, current wetting frequency, behavior problems that may be present, family history of enuresis, periods of previous dryness, other incontinent problems, parental reactions and degree of cooperation, and child's motivation for treatment.
2. Have a medical exam by a physician to rule out organic factors.
3. Encourage the child to take an active role in treatment. In taking the history direct the questions to the child and allow the parents to elaborate. Tell the child and the parents about the nature of the problem and give a rationale that does not find fault with the child. Repeatedly assure the child that he or she can be helped since suggestion is a potent force in the treatment of children. Give a brief explanation of the physiology of bladder functioning.
4. Warn the parents against a punitive approach to the problem. The use of shaming, threats, and spankings are useless and may be harmful. Such practices make the child anxious, embarrassed and unhappy. They frequently arouse negativism, resentment, and resistance to treatment. Ask the parents to be calm, patient and understanding about the problem and to limit themselves to supportive measures (praise, encouragement, reassurance and positive expectancy of success).

5. Assist the family to keep a record of progress which involves a nightly record of wetting incidents, size of wet spots, time wet and child's voiding on own at night.

6. Caution against restricting fluids at night. It is usually not beneficial since the bladder continues to empty periodically even if oral liquids are withheld for days, and this practice may delay or impede treatment.

7. Closely supervise the treatment program by daily telephone calls and periodic office visits. Failure to do so invites poor cooperation by the parents and child and, thus, an unfavorable outcome. The evidence shows that poor results are obtained when parents attempt to administer the bell and pad on their own without close supervision.

8. Therapists who expect the treatment to work and communicate this expectancy to the child and parents are more likely to achieve success.

FURTHER RESEARCH AND EXPERIMENTATION

Although substantial advances have been made in the treatment of enuresis over the last few decades, additional research is needed to corroborate the findings and uncover new approaches. More specifically, there is a pressing need for research in the following areas:

1. To further assess the validity and mode of action of different techniques.
2. To develop assessment procedures that could form the basis for the differential application of procedures.
3. To conduct long-term follow-ups (over one year in duration) of treatment effects.
4. To investigate the family characteristics of failure cases.
5. To compare specific toilet training practices of parents of enuretic vs nonenuretics.
6. To study the effectiveness of combining two or more interventions.
7. To assess the factors that influence the acceptability of treatment by parents and children.
8. To further study the effectiveness of less aversive forms of treatment such as the responsibility-reinforcement method and self-hypnosis.

Doleys (1977) suggests the following guidelines to make further research more comparable and interpretable:

"(a) The treatment procedure and apparatus should be clearly specified; (b) descriptive characteristics of the subject population and the wetting behavior should be given; (c) treatment should be carried out until a dryness or failure criterion is met and quantitative data collected; (d) follow-up data available with the initial report; and (e) relapses should be re-treated and quantitative data reported." (p. 51)

Glossary

anticholinergic. A drug that reduces bladder tone and the frequency and amplitude of bladder contractions.

bladder (urinary). The muscular, membranous, distensible reservoir for the urine. Innervated with nerves derived from the third and fourth sacral by way of the hypogastric plexus. It is situated in the anterior part of the pelvic cavity, in front of the anterior wall of the vagina and the uterus, and in the male, it lies in front of the rectum. It is about 5 x 3 x 5 inches in adult size and has a storage capacity of one-half to one pint, although it may be greatly distended.

cloaca. A toilet bowl.

cystitis. Inflammation of the bladder. Can result in frequent and painful urination in drops.

cystogram. X-ray film of the bladder.

cystoscope. Instrument for interior examination of bladder.

cystoscopy. Examination of the bladder with a cystoscope.

cystospasm. Spasmodic contractions of the urinary bladder.

cystoureterogram. A picture of the bladder and ureter.

detrusor (urinae). The external longitudinal layer of muscle coat around the bladder.

diuresis. An increased or excessive secretion or flow of urine.

diuretic. Increasing the secretion and flow of urine.

dysuria. Difficult or painful urination.

enuresis. Involuntary urination by a child four years old or older.

enuresis (primary or persistent). Child never had a substantial period of dry nights.

enuresis (secondary or acquired). Child had achieved nighttime control of bladder for at least one year but subsequently relapsed and resumed bedwetting. The cause of this is often a traumatic event.

enuresis ratio (ER). $\frac{\text{Number of wets}}{\text{Number of nights recorded.}}$ An ER of 1.00 indicates a wetting frequency averaging one wet per night.

heredity. The transmission from parent to offspring of certain characteristics.

irritable bladder. Marked by a constant desire to urinate.

kidney. One of two glandular, bean-shaped bodies, situated at the back of the abdominal cavity one on each side of the spinal column, which excrete waste matter in the form of urine.

micturate. To discharge urine from the body.

nephritis. Inflammation of the kidney.

nocturia. Excessive urination at night.

perineal. Of the perineum, i.e., the region of the body between the thighs, at the outlet of the pelvis.

placebo. A drug containing no medicine but given for its psychological effect.

polyuria. Excessive secretion and discharge of urine. Several hundred ounces a day may be voided by a child who has to go several times an hour.

pyuria. Pus in the urine; evidence of a kidney disease.

renal. Pertaining to the kidney.

somnambulism. The habit or act of sleepwalking, that is, getting up and moving about in a trancelike state while sleeping.

somniloquy. The habit or act of talking while asleep.

sphincter (bladder). Circular muscle constricting opening of bladder into urethra.

spinal dysraphism. Incomplete closure of the neural tube in the spinal cord.

strangury. Painful and interrupted urination in drops, produced by spasmodic muscular contraction of urethra and bladder. Often the result of cystitis.

uremia. Toxic condition caused by the presence in the blood of waste products normally eliminated in the urine; it results from an inadequate secretion of urine.

ureter. One of two tubes carrying urine from the kidneys to the bladder, beginning with the pelvis of the kidney, and emptying into the base of the bladder.

ureterography. X-ray photography of the ureter.

urethra. A canal for the discharge of urine extending from the bladder to the outside.

urethroscope. An instrument for examining the interior of the urethra.

urine. In mammals, the yellowish fluid containing urea and other waste products, secreted from the blood by the kidneys, passed down the ureters to the bladder, where it is stored, and periodically discharged from the body through the urethra.

void. To empty the bladder.

References

Abe, K, Shinakawa, M. and Kajiyama, S. Interaction between genetic and psychological factors in acquisition of bladder control in children. *Psychiatria et Neurologia,* 1967, **154**, 144–149.

Abelew, P.H. Intermittent schedules of reinforcement applied to the conditioning treatment of enuresis. *Dissentation Abstracts International,* 1972, **33**, 2799B–2800B.

Achenbach, T.M., and Lewis, M. A proposed model for clinical research and its application to encopresis and enuresis. *Journal of Child Psychiatry,* 1971, **10**, 535–554.

Ackerson, L. and Highlander, M. The relation of enuresis to intelligence, to conduct and personality problems, and to other factors. *Psychological Clinic,* 1928, **17**, 119–129.

Agarwala, S. and Heycock, J.B. A controlled trial of Imipramine (Tofranil) in the treatment of childhood enuresis. *British Journal of Clinical Practice,* 1968, **22**, 296–298.

Alderton, H.R. Imipramine in the treatment of nocturnal enuresis of childhood. *Canadian Psychiatric Association Journal,* 1965, **10**, 141–151.

Alderton, H.R. Imipramine in childhood nocturnal enuresis: Relationship of time of administration to effect. *Canadian Psychiatric Association Journal,* 1967, **12**, 197–203.

Allgeier, A.R. Minimizing therapist supervision in the treatment of enuresis. *Journal of Behavior Therapy and Experimental Psychiatry,* 1976, **7**, 371–372.

Altos, W.S. Some correlates of enuresis among illiterate soldiers. *Journal of Consulting Psychology,* 1946, **10**, 246–259.

Alvarez, W.C. Buzzer can help bedwetters. *Minneapolis Star.* December 2, 1970.

Amchin, A. Personality patterns of adolescent delinquent enuretics: A comparative analysis between adolescent delinquents who are known to be enuretic and adolescent delinquents who are known not to be enuretic. L.C. Card No. Mic 58–7613–New York University, 1958.

American Medical Assn. (Editorial) Nocturnal enuresis. *Journal of the American Medical Assn.,* 1954, **154** (6), 509.

Anders, T.F., and Weinstein, P. Sleep and its disorders in infants and children: A review. *Pediatrics,* 1974, **50,** 312–324.

Anderson, F.N. The psychiatric aspects of enuresis. *American Journal of the Diseases of Children,* 1930, **40,** 591–618; 818–850.

Arnold, S.J. Enuresis. *American Journal of the Diseases of Children,* 1972, **123,** 84.

Azrin, N.H. and Foxx, R.M. *Toilet training in less than a day.* New York, Simon and Schuster, 1974.

Azrin, N.H., Sneed, T.J. and Foxx, R.M. Dry-bed training: Rapid elimination of childhood enuresis. *Behaviour Research and Therapy,* 1974, **12,** 147–156.

Azrin, N.H. and Thienes, P.M. Rapid elimination of enuresis by intensive learning without a conditioning apparatus. *Behavior Therapy,* 1978, **9,** 342–354.

Bach, R. and Moylan, J.J. Parents administer behavior therapy for inappropriate urination and encopresis: A case study. *Journal of Behavior Therapy and Experimental Psychiatry,* 1975, **6,** 239–241.

Baker, B.L. Symptom treatment and symptom substitution in enuresis. *Journal of Abnormal Psychology,* 1969, **74,** 42–49.

Bakwin, H. Enuresis in children. *Journal of Pediatrics,* 1938, **12,** 757–768.

Bakwin, H. Sleep walking in twins. *Lancet,* 1970, **2,** 446.

Baller, W.R. *Bed-wetting: Origin and treatment.* New York, Pergamon, 1975.

Baller, W.R. and Giangreco, J.C. Correction of nocturnal enuresis in deaf children. *Volta Review,* 1970, **72** (9), 545–547.

Baller, W.R. and Schalock, H.D. Conditioned response treatment of enuresis. *Exceptional Children,* 1956, **22,** 233–236; 247–248.

Barclay, M. and Kubly, D. Results of treatment of enuresis by a conditioned response method. *Journal of Consulting Psychology,* 1955, **19,** 71–73.

Batty, R.J. *Enuresis or Bed-Wetting.* New York, Staples Press, 1948.

Behric, F.C., Elkin, M.T., Laybourne, P.C. Evaluation of a conditioning device in the treatment of nocturnal enuresis. *Pediatrics,* 1956, **17,** 849–855.

Benjamin, L.S., Serdahely, W., and Geppert, T.V. Night training through parents' implicit use of operant conditioning. *Child Development,* 1971, **42,** 963–966.

Benjamin, L.S., Stover, D.O., Geppert, T.V., Pizer, E.F., and Burdy, J. The relative importance of psychopathology, training procedure and urological pathology in nocturnal enuresis. *Child Psychiatry and Human Development,* 1971, **1,** 215–232.

Berezin, M.A. Enuresis and bisexual identification. *Journal of American Psychoanalysis Association,* 1954, **2,** 509–513.

Bettelheim, B. *The Children of the Dream.* London, Collier-MacMillan, 1969.

Bicknell, F. *Enuresis or bed-wetting,* London, Heinemann Press, 1959.

Biering, A. and Jesperson, I. The treatment of enuresis nocturna with conditioning devices. *Acta Paediatricia,* 1959, **118,** 152–153.

Bindelglas, P.M., Dee, G.H. and Enos, F.A. Medical and psychosocial factors in enuretic children treated with imipramine hydrochloride. *American Journal of Psychiatry,* 1968, **124,** (3), 125–130.

Blackwell, B. The psychopharmacology of nocturnal enuresis. Paper presented at Symposium on Enuresis, Newcastle, England, 1971.

Blackwell, B. and Curragh, J. The psychopharmacology of nocturnal enuresis. In Kalvin, I., MacKeith, R.C., and Meadow, S.R. (eds.), *Bladder Control and Enuresis,* London, England, S.I.M.P. with Heinemann Medical, 1973.

Bloomfield, J.M. and Douglas, J. Enuresis: Prevalence among children aged 4–7 years. *Lancet,* 1956, **1**, 850.

Bollard, R.J. and Woodroffe, P. The effect of parent-administered dry-bed training on nocturnal enuresis in children. *Behaviour Research and Therapy,* 1977, **15**, 159–165.

Borrie, P. and Fenton, J. Buzzer ulcers. *British Medical Journal,* 1966, **2**, 151.

Bostock, J. Enuresis and toilet training. *Medical Journal of Australia,* 1951, **1**, 110–113.

Bostock, J. and Shackleton, M. The enuresis dyad. *Medical Journal of Australia,* 1952, **2**, 356–360.

Bostock, J. and Shackleton, M. Maturation factor in enuresis. *Medical Journal of Australia,* 1956, **6**, 1042–1043.

Boyd, M.M. The depth of sleep in enuretic school children and in nonenuretic controls. *Journal of Psychosomatic Research,* 1960, **44**, 274–281.

Braithwaite, J.V. Problems connected with enuresis. President's address, *Proceedings of the Royal Society of Medicine,* 1956, **49**, 33–38.

Bransby, E.R., Blomfield, J.M. and Douglas, J.W.B. The prevalence of bed-wetting. *Medical Officer,* 1955, **94**, 5–7.

Brazelton, T.B. A child-oriented approach to toilet training. *Pediatrics,* 1962, **29**, 121–127.

Breckenridge, M.E. and Vincent, E.L. *Child Development: Physical and Psychological Growth Through Adolescence.* Philadelphia, Saunders, 1966.

Broughton, R.C. Sleep disorders: Disorders of arousal? *Science,* 1968, **159**, 1070–1078.

Brown, R.C. and Ford-Smith, A. Enuresis in adolescents. *British Medical Journal,* 1941, **2**, 803.

Browning, R.M. Operantly strengthening U.C.R. (awakening) as a prerequisite to treatment of persistent enuresis. *Behaviour Research and Therapy,* 1967, **5**, 371–372.

Butler, J.F. The toilet training success of parents after reading "Toilet training in less than a day." *Behavior Therapy,* 1976, **7**, 185–191.

Butler, J.F. Toilet training a child with Spina Befida. *Journal of Behavior Therapy and Experimental Psychiatry,* 1976b, **7**, 63–65.

Campbell, M.F. A clinical study of persistent enuresis. *New York State Journal of Medicine,* 1934, **34**, 190.

Campbell, M.F. Enuresis. *Archives of Pediatrics,* 1937, **54**, 187.

Campbell, M.F. *Clinical Pediatric Urology.* Philadelphia and London, Saunders, 1951, p. 848.

Campbell, M.F. Neuromuscular uropathy. In M.F. Campbell, and J.H. Harrison (eds.), *Urology,* **Vol. 2** Philadelphia, Saunders, 1970.

Catalina, D. Enuresis: Parent-mediated modification. Paper presented at the Eastern Psychological Association Convention, April, 1976.

Chamberlin, R.W. Management of preschool behavior problems. *Pediatric Clinics of North America,* 1974, **21**, 33–47.

Chapman, A.H. *Management of emotional problems in children and adolescents.* Philadelphia, Lippincott, 1974.

Ciminero, A.R. and Doleys, D.M. Childhood enuresis: Considerations in Assessment. *Journal of Pediatric Psychology,* 1976, **4**, 17–20.

Collins, D.R. Hypnotherapy in the management of nocturnal enuresis. *Medical Journal of Australia,* 1970, **1**, 52.

Collins, R.W. Importance of the bladder-cue buzzer contingency in the conditioning treatment for enuresis. *Journal of Abnormal Psychology,* 1973, **82**, 299–308.

Compton, R.D. Changes in enuretics accompanying treatment by the conditioned response technique. Unpublished doctoral dissertation. University of Nebraska, 1967.

Coote, M.A. Apparatus for conditioning treatment of enuresis. *Behaviour Research and Therapy,* 1965, **2**, 233–238.

Crandall, W. A method of treatment for nocturnal enuresis. *Journal of Clinical Psychology,* 1946, **2**, 175–178.

Creer, T.L. and Davis, M.H. Using a staggered-wakening procedure with enuretic children in an institutional setting. *Journal of Behavior Therapy and Experimental Psychiatry,* 1975, **6**, 23–25.

Crosby, N.D. Essential enuresis: Successful treatment based on physiological concepts. *Medical Journal of Australia,* 1953, **3**, 533–543.

Cushing, F.C. and Baller, W.R. The problem of nocturnal enuresis in adults: Special reference to managers and managerial aspirants. *Journal of Psychology,* 1976, **89**, 203–213.

Cust, G. The epidemiology of nocturnal enuresis. *Lancet,* 1958, **275**, 1167–1169.

Daniels, S.J. Enuresis: Body language and the positive aspects of the enuretic act. *American Journal of Psychotherapy,* 1971, **25**, 564–578.

Davidson, J.R. and Douglas, E. Nocturnal enuresis. *British Medical Journal,* 1950, **1**, 1345–1347.

DeLeon, G. and Mandell, W. A comparison of conditioning and psychotherapy in the treatment of functional enuresis. *Journal of Clinical Psychology,* 1966, **22**, 326–330.

DeLeon, G. and Sacks, S. Conditioning functional enuresis: A four-year follow-up. *Journal of Consulting and Clinical Psychology,* 1972, **39**, 299–300.

DeLuca, J. Psychosexual conflict in adolescent enuretics. *Journal of Psychology,* 1968, **70**, 145–149.

Dement, W.C. and Guilleminault, C. Sleep disorders: The state of the art. *Hospital Practice,* 1973, **8**, 57–71.

Despert, J. Urinary control and enuresis. *Psychosomatic Medicine,* 1944, **6**, 294–307.

Dewdney, J.C. and Dewdney, M.S. Wake them at night: Incidence of nocturnal enuresis amoung a group of institutionalized boys: Effect of a space arousal program. *Child Care Quarterly Review,* 1965, **19**, 96–101.

Dibden, W.A. and Holmes, M.A. Enuresis, a survey of its treatment by the "dri-nite" apparatus. *Clinical Reports* (Adelaide Children's Hospital), 1955, **2**, 247–255.

Dimson, S.B. Toilet training and enuresis. *British Medical Journal,* 1959, **2**, 666–670.

DiPerry, R. and Medurri, M. L'enuresi notturna: Ulteriori elementi in tema di diagnostica strumentale. *Acta Neurology,* (Napoli), 1972, **27**, 22–27.

Dische, S. Management of enuresis. *British Medical Journal,* 1971, **2**, 33–36.

Dische, S. Treatment of enuresis with an enuresis alarm. In I. Kolvin, R.C. MacKeith, and S.R. Meadow (eds.) *Bladder Control and enuresis.* Philadelphia, Pa., Lippincott, 1973.

Dittman, K.S. and Blinn, K.A. Sleep levels in enuresis. *American Journal of Psychiatry,* 1955, **12**, 913–920.

Doleys, D.M. Behavioral treatments for nocturnal enuresis in children. A review of the recent literature. *Psychological Bulletin,* 1977, **84**, 30–54.

Doleys, D.M. and Ciminero, A.R. Childhood enuresis: Consideration in treatment, *Journal of Pediatric Psychology,* 1976, **4**, 21–23.

Doleys, D.M., Ciminero, A.R., Tollison, J.W., Williams, C.L. and Wells, K.C. Dry-bed training and retention control training: A comparison. *Behavior Therapy,* 1977, **8**, 541–548.

Doleys, D.M. and Wells, K.C. Changes in functional bladder capacity and bed-wetting during and after retention control training: A case study. *Behavior Therapy,* 1975, **6**, 685–688.

Dollard, J. and Miller, N.E. *Personality and Psychotherapy.* New York, McGraw-Hill, 1950, p. 136.

Douglas, J.W. Early disturbing events and later enuresis. In I. Kolvin, R.C. MacKeith and S.R. Meadows (eds.), *Bladder Control and Enuresis,* London, Heinemann, 1973.

Edwardsen, P. Neurophysiological aspects of enuresis. *Acta Neurologica Scandinavia,* 1972, **48**, 222–230.

Ellis, N.R. Toilet training the severely defective patient: An S.R. reinforcement analysis. *American Journal of Mental Deficiency,* 1963, **68**, 98–103.

Ellison-Nash, D.F. The development of micturition control with special reference to enuretics. *Annals of the Royal College of Surgeons,* England, 1949, **5**, 318.

English, O.S. and Pearson, G.H. *Emotional Problems of Living,* New York, Norton, 1945.

Epstein, S.J. and Guilfoyle, F.M. Imipramine (Tofranil) in the control of enuresis. *American Journal of the Diseases of Children,* 1965, **109**, 412–415.

Evans, J.W. The etiology and treatment of enuresis. *Journal of Pediatrics,* 1937, **11**, 683–690.

Faschingbauer, T.R. Enuresis: Its nature, etiology, and treatment: A review of the literature, 1924–1970. *JSAS Catalog of Selected Documents for Psychology,* 1975, **5**, 194.

Finley, W.W., Besserman, R.L., Bennett, L.F., Clapp, R.K. and Finley, P.M. The effect of continuous intermittent and "placebo" reinforcement on the effectiveness of the conditioning treatment for enuresis nocturna. *Behaviour Research and Therapy,* 1973, **11**, 289–297.

Finley, W.W. and Smith, H.A. A long-life, inexpensive urine-detection pad for conditioning of enuresis nocturna. *Behavior Research Methods and Instruments,* 1975, **7**, 273–276.

Finley, W.W. and Wansley, R.A. Use of intermittent reinforcement in a clinical-research program for the treatment of enuresis nocturna. *Journal of Pediatric Psychology,* 1976, **4**, 24–27.

Finley, W.W. and Wansley, R.A. Auditory intensity as a variable in the conditioning treatment of enuresis nocturna. *Behaviour Research and Therapy,* 1977, **15**, 181–185.

Fleisher, D.R. Diagnosis and treatment of disorders of defecation in children. *Pediatric Gastroenterology,* 1976, **87**, 700–722.

Forrester, R.M., Stein, Z. and Susser, M.W. A trial of conditioning therapy in nocturnal enuresis. *Developmental Medicine and Child Neurology,* 1964, **6**, 158–166.

Forsythe, W.I., and Merrett, J.D. A controlled trial of Imipramine (Tofranil) and Nortriptyline (Allegron) in the treatment of enuresis. *British Journal of Clinical Practice,* 1969, **23**, 210.

Forsythe, W.I., Redmond, A. Enuresis and the electric alarm study of 200 cases. *British Medical Journal,* 1970, **1**, 211.

Forsythe, W.I. and Redmond, A. Enuresis and spontaneous cure rate. *Archives of Diseases of Childhood,* 1974, **49**, 259.

Foxx, R.M. and Azrin, N.H. Dry pants: A rapid method of toilet training children. *Behaviour Research and Therapy,* 1973 (a), **11**, 435–442.

Foxx, R.M. and Azrin, N.H. *Toilet training the retarded: A rapid program for day and nighttime independent toileting.* Champaign, Ill.: Research Press, 1973 (b).

Frary, L.G. Enuresis: A genetic study. *American Journal of the Diseases of Children,* 1935, **49**, 557–578.

Freeman, E.D. The treatment of enuresis: An overview. *International Journal of Psychiatry in Medicine,* 1975, **6**, 403–412.

Freyman, R. Follow-up study of enuresis treated with a bell apparatus. *Journal of Child Psychology and Psychiatry,* 1963, **4**, 199–266.

Fried, R. A device for enuresis control. *Behavior Therapy,* 1974, **5**, 682–683.

Friedell, A. A reversal of the normal concentration of the urine in children having enuresis. *American Journal of the Diseases of Children,* 1927, **33**, 717–721.

Friedman, A.R. Behavior training in a case of enuresis. *Journal of Individual Psychology,* 1968, **24**, 86–87.

Galdston, R., and Perlmutter, A.D. The urinary manifestations of anxiety in children. *Pediatrics,* 1973, **52**, 818–822.

Gedda, L., Alfieri, A., Bronchi, G., Reggiani, L. and Lun, M.T. Primary enuresis studied by the twin method. *Acta Geniticoa Medicae et Gemillologiae,* 1970, **19**, 258–260.

Genouville, L. Incontinence L'urine. *L'association Francaise d'urologie,* 1908, **12**, 97.

Geppert, T.V. Management of nocturnal enuresis by conditioned response. *Journal of the American Medical Association,* 1953, **152**, 381-383.

Gerard, M.W. Child analysis as a technique in the investigation of mental mechanisms. *Journal of Psychiatry,* 1937, **74**, 652-663.

Gerard, M.W. *The emotionally disturbed child.* New York, Child Welfare, 1959.

Gerrard, J.W. Allergy and urinary infections: Is there an association? *Pediatrics,* 1971, **48**, 994.

Glicklich, L.B. A historical account of enuresis. *Pediatrics,* 1951, **8**, 859-876.

Gillison, T.H. and Skinner, J.L. Treatment of nocturnal enuresis by electric alarm. *British Medical Journal,* 1958, **2**, 1268-1273.

Granata, M., and Piazza, M. Sull enuresi nocturna: Contributo-clinica electroenfaligrafico e terapeutico. *Rivista di Neuro-biologia,* 1967, **13 (4)**, 900-919.

Greaves, M.W. Hazards of enuresis alarm. *Archives of Diseases of Childhood,* 1969, **44**, 285-286.

Gunnarson, S. and Melin, K.A. The electroencephalogram in enuresis. *Acta Pediatricia,* 1951, **40**, 496-501.

Hagglund, T.B. Enuretic children treated with fluid restriction or forced drinking. *Annuals of Paedriatrica,* 1965, **11**, 84.

Hallgren, B. Enuresis: A study with reference to certain physical, mental and social factors possibly associated with enuresis. *Acta Psychiatriet Neurologica Scandinavia,* 1956, **31**, 405-436.

Hallgren, B. Enuresis: A clinical and genetic study. *Acta Psychiatriet Neurologica Scandinavia,* 1957, **32 (114)**, 1-59.

Hallman, N. On the ability of enuretic children to hold urine. *Acta Paediatrica,* 1950, **39**, 87.

Hamil, R.C. Enuresis. *Journal of the American Medical Association,* 1962, **49 (1)**, 979-980.

Harris, D.H. Are enuretics suitable for the armed forces? *Journal of clinical Psychology,* 1957, **1 (13)**, 91-93.

Harris, L.S. Bladder training and enuresis. *Behaviour Research and Therapy,* 1977, **15**, 485-490.

Hawkins, D.N. Enuresis: A survey. *Medical Journal of Australia,* 1962, **49**, 979-980.

Hicks, W.R. and Barnes, E.H. A double blind study of the effect of Imipramine on enuresis in 100 naval recruits. *American Journal of Psychiatry,* 1964, **120**, 812.

Hodge, R.S. and Hutchins, H.M. Enuresis: A brief review, a tentative theory and a suggested treatment. *Archives of Diseases of Childhood,* 1952, **27**, 498-504.

Holt, K.S. Drug treatment of enuresis: Controlled trials with brobantheline, amphetamine and pituitary snuff. *Lancet,* 1956, **2**, 1334-1336.

Homan, W.E. *Child sense: A guide to loving, level-headed parenthood.* New York, Basic Books, 1977.

Hundziak, M., Maurer, R.A. and Watson, L.S. Operant conditioning in toilet training of severely mentally retarded boys. *American Journal of Mental Deficiency,* 1965, **70**, 120–124.

Huschka, M. The child's response to coercive bowel training. *Psychosomatic Medicine,* 1942, **4**, 301–308.

James, L.E. and Foreman, M.E. A-B status of behavior therapy technicians as related to success of Mowrer's conditioning treatment for enuresis. *Journal of Consulting and Clinical Psychology,* 1973, **41**, 224–229.

Jehu, D., Morgan, R. T.T., Turner, R.K., and Jones, A. A controlled trial of the treatment of nocturnal enuresis in residential homes for children. *Behaviour Research and Therapy,* 1977, **15**, 1–16.

Johnson, S.H. and Marshall, M. Enuresis. *Journal of Urology,* 1954, **71**, 554–559.

Jones, H.G. The behavioral treatment of enuresis nocturna. In Eysenck, H.J. (ed.), *Behaviour therapy and the neuroses,* Oxford, England, Pergamon, 1960.

Kahane, M. An experimental investigation of a conditioning treatment; and a preliminary study of the psychoanalytic theory of etiology of nocturnus enuresis. *American Psychologist,* 1955, **10**, 369–370.

Kales, J.D., Jacobson, A., and Kales, A. Sleep disorders in children. *Progress in Clinical Pathology,* 1968, **8**, 63.

Kardash, S., Hillman, E.S. and Werry, J. Efficacy of Imipramine in childhood enuresis, a double-blind control study with placebo. *Canadian Medical Association Journal,* 1968, **99**, 263–266.

Katz, J. Enuresis and encopresis. *Medical Journal of Australia,* 1972, **1**, 127–130.

Kempe, C.H. and Helfer, R.E. *Helping the battered child and his family.* Oxford, England, Lippincott, 1972.

Kennedy, W.A. and Sloop, E.W. Methedrine as an adjunct to conditioning treatment of nocturnal enuresis in normal and institutionalized retarded subjects. *Psychological Reports,* 1968, **22**, 997–1000.

Kimmel, H.D. Review of "Toilet training in less than a day." *Journal of Behavior Therapy and Experimental Psychiatry,* 1974, **5**, 113–114.

Kimmel, H.D. and Kimmel, E. An instrumental conditioning method for the treatment of enuresis. *Journal of Behavior Therapy and Experimental Psychiatry,* 1970, **1**, 121–123.

Klackenberg, G. Primary enuresis: When is child dry at night? *Acta Paediatrica,* 1955, **44**, 513.

Kolvin, J., Fauch, J., Garside, R.F., Nolan, J., and Shaw, W.B. Enuresis: A descriptive analysis and a controlled trial. *Developmental Medicine and Child Neurology,* 1972, **14**, 715–726.

Kraus, J., Keil, J. and Isles, J.C. On the treatment of enuresis. *Medical Journal of Australia,* 1962, **1**, 511–512.

Kriegman, G., and Wright, H.B. Brief psychotherapy with enuretics in the Army. *American Journal of Psychiatry,* 1947, **104**, 254–258.

Kroger, W.S. *Clinical and Experimental Hypnosis.* Philadelphia, Lippincott, 1963.

Labay, P. and Boyarsky, S. The pharmacology of Imipramine and its mechanism of action on enuresis. *Archives of Physical Medicine and Rehabilitation,* 1972, **53**, 584.

Lasar, P. L'enuresis nocturne chez l'enfant, premiers lssais d'un traitement base sur le neuraphysiologie du sommeil. *Acta Urologica et Psychiatric Belgico,* 1965, **65**, 127–133.

Levine, A. Enuresis in the Navy. *American Journal of Psychiatry,* 1943, **100**, 320–325.

Lickorish, J.R. One hundred enuretics. *Journal of Psychology,* 1963, **7**, 263–267.

Litrownik, A.J. A method for home training an incontinent child. *Journal of Behavior Therapy and Experimental Psychiatry,* 1974, **5**, 77–80.

Linderholm, B.E. The cystometric findings in enuresis. *Journal of Urology,* 1966, **96**, 718–722.

Lobrot, M. Etude des enfants enuretique. *Enfance,* 1963, **3**, 209–231.

Lovibond, S.H. The mechanism of conditioning treatment of enuresis. *Behaviour Research and Therapy,* 1963a, **1**, 17–21.

Lovibond, S.H. Positive and negative conditioning of the G.S.R. *Acta Psycholico,* 1963b, **21**, 106–107.

Lovibond, S.H. Intermittent reinforcement in behavior therapy. *Behaviour Research and Therapy,* 1963c, **1**, 127–132.

Lovibond, S.H. *Conditioning and Enuresis,* New York, Pergamon Press, 1964.

Lovibond, S.H. and Coote, M.A. Enuresis In C.G. Costello (ed.), *Symptoms of Psychopathology,* New York, Wiley, 1970.

MacKeith, R.C. A frequent factor in the origins of primary nocturnal enuresis: Anxiety in the third year of life. *Developmental Medicine and Child Neurology,* 1968, **10**, 465–470.

MacKeith, R.C. Is maturation delay a frequent factor in the origins of primary nocturnal enuresis? *Developmental Medicine and Child Neurology,* 1972, **14**, 217–223.

Maclean, R.E.G. Imipramine hydrochloride (Tofranil) and enuresis. *American Journal of Psychiatry,* 1960, **117**, 551.

Mahoney, D. Incidence of obstructive lesions and pathophysiology of enuresis. *Journal of Urology,* 1971, **106**, 951.

Marshall, S., Marshall, H.H., and Lyon, R.P. Enuresis: An analysis of various therapeutic approaches. *Pediatrics,* 1973, **52**, 813–817.

Martin, B. and Kubly, D. Results of treatment of enuresis by a conditioned response method. *Journal of Consulting Psychology,* 1955, **19**, 71–73.

Martin, G.L. Imipramine promate in the treatment of childhood enuresis: A double blind study. *New York State Journal of Medicine,* 1971, **122**, 42–47.

Martin, G.I. and Zaug, P.J. ECG monitoring of enuretic children given Imipramine. *Journal of the American Medical Association,* 1973, **223**, 902–903.

Matson, J.L. Some practical considerations for using the Foxx and Azrin rapid method of toilet training. *Psychological Reports,* 1975, **37**, 350.

Matson, J.L. and Ollendick, T.H. Issues in toilet training normal children. *Behavior Therapy,* 1977, **8**, 549–553.

Mayon-White, R.M. A controlled trial of Propantheline in bed-wetting. *British Medical Journal,* 1926, **1**, 550.

McConaghy, N. A controlled trial of Imipramine, Amphetamine, pad-and-bell conditioning and random awakening in the treatment of nocturnal enuresis. *Medical Journal of Australia,* 1969, **2**, 237–239.

McKendry, J.B., Williams, H.A. and Matheson, D. Enuresis: A three year study of the value of a waking apparatus. *Canadian Medical Association Journal,* 1964, **90**, 513–516.

McKendry, J.B., Stewart, D.A., Jeffs, R.D., and Mozes, A. Enuresis treated by improved waking apparatus. *Canadian Medical Association Journal,* 1972, **106**, 27–29.

McLellan, F.C. *The neurogenic bladder.* Springfield, Ill., Thomas, 1939.

Meadow, R. Childhood enuresis. *British Medical Journal,* 1970, **4**, 787–789.

Meadow, R. Drugs for bed-wetting. *Archives of Diseases of Childhood,* 1974, **49**, 257.

Meadow, S.R. Buzzer ulcers. In I. Kolvin, R.C. MacKeith, and S.R. Meadow (eds.), *Bladder Control and Enuresis;* Philadelphia, Lippincott, 1973.

Mesibov, O.B., Schroeder, C.S. and Wesson, L. Parental concerns about their children. *Journal of Pediatric Psychology,* 1977, **2**, 13–17.

Michaels, J.J. Disorders of character: Persistent enuresis, juvenile delinquency and psychopathic personality. *Archives of Neurology and Psychiatry,* 1954, **72**, 641–643.

Michaels, J.J. Enuresis in murderous aggressive children and adolescents. *Archives of General Psychiatry,* 1964, **10**, 490–493.

Michaels, J.H. and Goodman, S.E. Incidence and inter-correlations of enuresis and other neuropathic traits in so-called normal child. *American Journal of Orthopsychiatry,* 1934, **4**, 79–106.

Miller, P.M. An experimental analysis of retention control training in the treatment of nocturnal enuresis in two institutionalized adolescents. *Behavior Therapy,* 1973, **4**, 288–294.

Miller, P.R., Champelli, J.W. and Dinelio, F.A. Imipramine in the treatment of enuretic school children. A double-blind study. *American Journal of Disorders of Childhood,* 1968, **115**, 17.

Morgan, J.B., and Witmer, F.J. The treatment of enuresis by the conditioned reaction technique. *Journal of Genetic Psychology,* 1939, **5**, 59–65.

Morgan, R.T.T., and Young, G.C. The conditioning treatment of childhood enuresis. *British Journal of Social Work,* 1972a, **2**, 503–509.

Morgan, R.T.T., and Young, G.C. The treatment of enuresis: Merits of conditioning methods. *Community Medicine,* 1972b, **128**, 119–121.

Morgan, R.T.T., and Young, G.C. Parental attitude and the conditioning treatment of childhood enuresis. *Behaviour Research and Therapy,* 1975, **13**, 197–199.

Mowrer, O.H. Apparatus for the study and treatment of enuresis. *American Journal of Psychology,* 1933, **51**, 163–166.

Mowrer, O.H. and Mowrer, W.M. Enuresis: A method for its study and treatment. *American Journal of Orthopsychiatry,* 1938, **8**, 436–459.

Muellner, S.R. The voluntary control of micturition in man. *Journal of Urology,* 1958, **80**, 473-478.

Muellner, S.R. Development of urinary control in children: A new concept in cause, prevention and treatment of primary enuresis. *Journal of Urology,* 1960, **84**, 714-716.

Muellner, S.R. Primary enuresis in children. *Biochemical Clinic,* 1963, **2**, 161.

Munster, A.J., Stanley, A.M. and Saunders, J.C. Imipramine (Tofranil) in the treatment of enuresis. *American Journal of Psychiatry,* 1961, **118**, 76-77.

Neal, B.W. and Coote, M.A. Hazards of enuresis alarms. *Archives of Diseases of Children,* 1969, **44**, 651.

Nichols, L.A. Enuresis: Its background and cure. *Lancet,* 1956, **271**, 1336-1337.

Nordquist, V.M. The modification of a child's enuresis: Some response-response relationships. *Journal of Applied Behavior Analysis,* 1971, **4**, 241-247.

Novick, J. Symptomatic treatment of acquired and persistent enuresis. *Journal of Abnormal Psychology,* 1966, **77**, 363-368.

Olness, K. The use of self-hypnosis in the treatment of childhood nocturnal enuresis. *Clinical Pediatrics,* 1975, **14**, 273-277.

Olness, K. How to help the wet child and the frustrated parents. *Modern Medicine,* 1977, September 30, 42-46.

Oppel, W.C. The age of attaining bladder control. *Pediatrics,* 1968, **42**, 614-626.

Oppel, W.C., Harper, P.A. and Rider, R.V. Social, psychological and neurological factors associated with nocturnal enuresis. *Pediatrics,* 1968, **42**, 627-641.

Parkin, J.M., and Fraser, M.S. Poisoning as a complication of enuresis. *Developmental Medicine and Child Neurology,* 1972, **44**, 727-730.

Paschalis, A.P., Kimmel, H.D., and Kimmel, E. Further study of diurnal instrumental conditioning in the treatment of enuresis nocturna. *Journal of Behavior Therapy and Experimental Psychiatry,* 1972, **3**, 253-256.

Petersen, K.E. and Anderson, O.O. Treatment of nocturnal enuresis with Imipramine and related preparations: A double blind trial with a placebo. *Acta Paedritria,* 1971, **60**, 244.

Peterson, R.A. The natural development of nocturnal bladder control. *Developmental Medicine and Child Neurology,* 1971, **13**, 730-734.

Peterson, R.A., Hanlon, C.C. and Wright, R.L.D. An evaluation of the conditioning process in the conditioning treatment of nocturnal enuresis. Paper presented at the Convention of the Society for Research in Child Development, 1967, New York.

Peterson, R.A., Wright, R.L.D., and Hanlon, C.C. The effects of extending the CS-UCS interval on the effectiveness of the conditioning treatment of nocturnal enuretics. *Behaviour Research and Therapy,* 1969, **7**, 351-357.

Pfaundler, M. Demonstration of an apparatus for automatic warning of the occurrence of bedwetting. *Verhandlungen der Gesellschaft fur Kinderheilpundl,* 1904, **21**, 219-220.

Pierce, C.M., Lipcan, H.H., McLary, J.H., and Nobel, H.F. Enuresis: Psychiatric interview studies. *United States Armed Forces Medical Journal,* 1956, **7**, (9), 1-12.

Pierce, C.M., Whitman, R., Maas, J. and Gay, M. Enuresis and dreaming: Experimental studies. *Archives of General Psychiatry,* 1961, **4**, 166–170.

Plag, J.A. The problem of enuresis in the Naval service. Report No. 64–3, US Navy Medical Neuropsychiatric Research Unit, San Diego, Ca. 1964.

Popler, K. Token reinforcement in the treatment of nocturnal enuresis: A case study and six month follow-up. *Journal of Behavior Therapy and Experimental Psychiatry,* 1976, **7**, 83–84.

Poulton, E.M. and Hinden, E., The classification of enuresis. *Archives of the Diseases of Children,* 1953, **28**, 392–397.

Poissaint, A.F. and Ditman, K.S. A controlled study of Imipramine (Tofranil) in the treatment of childhood enuresis. *Journal of Pediatrics,* 1965, **67**, 283–290.

Powell, N.B. Urinary incontinence in children. *Archives of Pediatrics,* 1951, **68**, 151–157.

Reid, W.B. Some aspects of personality in persistent enuresis as determined by responses to psychological tests and to drug therapy. Unpublished doctoral dissertation, University of Houston, 1966.

Remy-Roux C. Nouvel Appareil électrique contre l'incontinence nocturne d'urine. *Bulletins et memoires de la Société de médicine de Vaucluse, Avignon,* 1908–1911, **2**, 337.

Robb, E.R. Enuresis. *Minnesota Medicine,* 1947, **30**, 91–98.

Roberiello, R.C. Some psychic interrelations between the urinary and sexual systems with special reference to enuresis. *Psychiatric Quarterly,* 1956, **30**, 61–62.

Roberts, K.E., and Schoellkopf, R. Eating, sleeping and elimination practices of a group of 2 ½ year old children. *American Journal of Diseases of Children,* 1951, **82**, 121–126.

Romberger, J.A., *et al.* Psychosocial correlates of nocturnal enuresis. *Canadian Journal of Public Health,* 1977, **68**, 499–502.

Ross, J.A. Behavioral treatment of enuresis: Case study. *Psychological Reports,* 1974, **35**, 286.

Rutter, M., Yule, W. and Graham, P. Enuresis and behavioral deviance. In I. Kolvin, R.C. MacKeith, and S.R. Meadow (eds.), *Bladder Control and Enuresis,* London, Heinemann, 1973.

Sacks, S., and DeLeon, G. Conditioning of two types of enuretics. *Behaviour Research and Therapy,* 1973, **11**, 653–654.

Sadler, O.W. and Merkert, F. Evaluating the Foxx and Azrin toilet training procedure for retarded children in a day training center. *Behavior Therapy,* 1977, **8**, 499–500.

Samaan, M. The control of nocturnal enuresis by operant conditioning. *Behavior Therapy and Experimental Psychiatry,* 1972, **3**, 103–105.

Schachter, M. and Cotte, S. Les enfants enuretiques, *Zeitschrift Fues Kinderpsychiatric,* 1941, **8**, 102.

Schachter, M. and Cotte, S. Le problems des enuresies prolongs des adolescents. *Encephole,* 1968, **57** (**4**) 367–379.

Schauffler, G. Enuresis. *Urologic and Cutaneous Review,* 1942, **46**, 294–299.

Schiff, S.K. The E.E.G. eye movements and dreaming in adult enuresis, *Journal of Nervous and Mental Disease,* 1965, **140** (6). 379-404.

Schwartz, M.S., Colligan, R.C. and O'Connell, E.J. Behavior modification of nocturnal enuresis: A treatment and research program at the Mayo Clinic. *Professional Psychology,* 1972, Spring, 169-172.

Schwidder, W. (The hypnoanalytic treatment of a juvenile bedwetter) *Praxis de Kinderpsychologie und Kinderpsychiatric,* 1953, 2, 10-15.

Scoe, H.F. Bladder control in infancy and early childhood. *University of Iowa Studies in Child Welfare,* 1933, **5, No. 4,** Iowa City, Iowa.

Sears, R.R., Maccoby, E.E. and Levin, H. *Patterns of Child Rearing,* New York, Harper and Row, 1957.

Seiger, H.W. A practical urine or wet diaper signal. *Journal of Pediatrics,* 1946, **28,** 733.

Seiger, H.W. Treatment of essential nocturnal enuresis. *Journal of Pediatrics,* 1952, **40,** 738-749.

Shaffer, D., Costello, A.J., and Hill, I.D. Control of enuresis with Imipramine. *Archives of Diseases of Childhood,* 1968, **43,** 665-671.

Shaffer, D. Enuresis. *Update,* 1970, **2,** 725-726.

Sheldon, W. Discussion on enuresis, *Proceedings of the Royal Society of Medicine,* 1944, **37,** 348-349.

Shepherd, G. and Durham, R. The multiple techniques approach to behavioral psychotherapy: A retrospective evaluation of effectiveness and an examination of prognostic indicators. *British Journal of Medicine Psychology,* 1977, **50,** 45-52.

Shultz, F.W. and Anderson, C.E. Endocrine treatment of enuresis. *Journal of Clinical Endocrinology,* 1943, **3,** 407.

Silberstein, R.M. Enuresis: A controversial problem in child psychiatry. *Child Welfare,* 1973, **52,** 367-374.

Singh, R., Phillips, D. and Fischer, S.C. The treatment of enuresis by progressively earlier wakening. *Journal of Behavior Therapy and Experimental Psychiatry,* 1976, **7,** 277-278.

Smith, S. *The psychological origin and treatment of enuresis.* Seattle: University of Washington Press, 1948.

Smith, S. *Bedwetting: Its cause, effect, and remedy.* Valley Stream, N.Y., H.R. Press, 1974.

Solvey, G. and Milechnin, A. Concerning the treatment of enuresis. *American Journal of Clinical Hypnosis,* 1959, **2,** 22-30.

Sperling, M. Dynamic considerations and treatment of enuresis. *Journal of the American Academy of Child Psychiatry,* 1965, **4,** 19-31.

Spock, B. and Bergen, M. Parents' fear of conflict in toilet training. *Pediatrics,* 1964, **34,** 112-116.

Stalker, H. and Rand, D. Persistent enuresis: A psychosomatic study. *Journal of Mental Science,* 1946, **92,** 324-342.

Starfield, B. Functional bladder capacity in enuretic and nonenuretic children. *Journal of Pediatrics,* 1967, **70,** 771-781.

Starfield, B. and Mellits, E.D. Increase in functional bladder capacity and improvements in enuresis. *Journal of Pediatrics,* 1968, **72**, 483-487.

Stebbens, J.A. Enuresis in school children. *Journal of School Psychology,* 1970, **8**, 145-151.

Stedman, J.M. An extension of the Kimmel treatment method for enuresis to an adolescent: A case report. *Journal of Behavior Therapy and Experimental Psychiatry,* 1972, **3**, 307-309.

Stein, Z.A., and Susser, M.W. Nocturnal enuresis as a phenomenon of institutions. *Developmental Medicine and Child Neurology,* 1966, **8**, 677-685.

Stein, Z.A. and Susser, M.W. Social factors in the development of sphincter control. *Developmental Medicine and Child Neurology,* 1967, **9**, 692-706.

Stewart, C.B. Enuresis. *Canadian Medical Association Journal,* 1946, **55**, 370-372.

Stewart, M.A. Treatment of bedwetting. *Journal of The American Medical Association,* 1975, **232**, 281-283.

Stockwell, L. and Smith, C.K. Enuresis: A study of causes, types and therapeutic results. *American Journal of Diseases of Childhood,* 1940, **59**, 1013-1033.

Stokvis, B. Group psychotherapy of enuretic children by psychodrama and sociodrama. *American Journal of Psychotherapy,* 1954, **8 (1)**, 265-275.

Strom-Olsen, R. Enuresis in adults and abnormality of sleep. *Lancet,* 1950, **2**, 133-135.

Tabarka, K., Naglova, R., and Hribal, R. Our experiences with diadynamic currents in enuretic children. *Ceskoslovenska Psychiatric,* 1966, **62 (3)**, 193-196.

Takeuchi, M. Trial of an apparatus for the treatment of nocturnia and results of its use. *Journal of Therapy (Tokyo),* 1961, **43**, 2183-2187.

Tapia, F., Jekel, J. and Domke, H. Enuresis: An emotional symptom. *Journal of Nervous and Mental Disorder,* 1960, **130**, 61.

Taylor, I.O. A scheme for the treatment of enuresis by electric buzzer apparatus. *Medical Officer,* 1963, **110**, 130-140.

Taylor, P.D. and Turner, R.K. A clinical trial of continuous, intermittent and overlearning "Bell and Pad" treatment for nocturnal enuresis. *Behaviour Research and Therapy,* 1975, **13**, 281-293.

Tec, L. Imipramine as a treatment for enuretic children. *American Journal of Psychiatry,* 1964, **121**, 87.

Thomsen, W.V., Reid, W.B. and Hebeler, J. Effect of Tofranil on enuretic boys. *Diseases of the Nervous System,* 1967, **28 (3)**, 167-169.

Teichman, Y., *et al.* Overt and fantasized aggression towards parents by enuretic and nonenuretic children. *Journal of Abnormal Child Psychology,* 1977, **5**, 379-386.

Thomason, C.F. Correction of nocturnal enuresis in economically disadvantaged children. Unpublished Doctoral Dissertation, United States International University, 1971.

Thorne, D.E. Instrumental counterconditioning of enuresis with minimal therapist intervention. *Proceedings of the 81st Annual Convention of the American Psychological Association,* 1973, **8**, 451–452.

Thorne, D.E. Instrumental behavior modification of bedwetting. *Behavioral Engineering,* 1975, **2**, 47–51.

Thorne, F.C. The incidence of nocturnal enuresis after the age of five. *American Journal of Psychiatry,* 1944, **100**, 668–689.

Tough, J.H., Hawkins, R.P., MacArthur, M.M. and Ravensway, S.V. Modification of enuretic behavior by punishment: A new use for an old device. *Behavior Therapy,* 1971, **2**, 567–574.

Troup, C.W., and Hodgson, N.B. Nocturnal functional bladder capacity of enuretic children. *Pediatric Urology,* 1971, **105**, 129–132.

Turner, R.K. Conditioning treatment of nocturnal enuresis. In I. Kolvin, R.C. MacKeith, and S.R. Meadow (eds.), *Bladder Control and Enuresis.* Philadelphia, Lippincott, 1973.

Turner, R.K. and Taylor, R.D. Conditioning treatment of nocturnal enuresis in adults: Preliminary findings. *Behaviour Research and Therapy,* 1974, **12 (1)**, 41–52.

Turner, R.K., Rachman, S. and Young, G.C. Conditioning treatment of enuresis: A rejoinder to Lovibond. *Behaviour Research and Therapy,* 1972, **10**, 291–292.

Turner, R.K. and Young, G.C. CNS stimulant drugs and conditioning treatment of nocturnal enuresis: A long-term follow-up study. *Behaviour Research and Therapy,* 1966, **4**, 225–228.

Turner, R.K., Young, G.C. and Rachman, S. Treatment of nocturnal enuresis by conditioning techniques. *Behaviour Research and Therapy,* 1970, **8**, 367–381.

Turton, E.C., and Spear, A.B. EEG findings in 100 cases of severe enuresis. *Archives of Diseases of Childhood,* 1953, **28**, 316–320.

Vincent, S.A. The mechanism of bladder control. *Ulster Medical Journal,* 1959, **28**, 176–187.

Vincent, S.A. Treatment of enuresis with a perineal pressure apparatus: The irritable bladder syndrome. *Developmental Medicine and Child Neurology,* 1964, **6**, 23–31.

Vincent, S.A. Postural control of urinary incontinence. *Lancet,* 1966 (a), **6**, 631–632.

Vincent, S.A. Some aspects of bladder mechanisms. *Bio-Medical Engineering,* 1966b, **1**, 438–445.

Wadsworth, M.L. Persistent enuresis in adults, *American Journal of Orthopsychiatry,* 1944, **14**, 313–321.

Walker, C.E. Toilet training, enuresis and encopresis. In P.R. Magrab (ed.), *Psychological management of pediatric problems.* **Vol. I.** Baltimore, University Park Press, 1978.

Werry, J.S. Enuresis—a psychosomatic entity? *Canadian Medical Association Journal,* 1967, **97**, 319–327.

Werry, J.S. The conditioning treatment of enuresis. *American Journal of Psychiatry,* 1966, **123**, 226–229.

Werry, J.S. and Cohrssen, J. Enuresis: An etiologic and therapeutic study. *Journal of Pediatrics,* 1965, **67**, 423–431.

Wexberg, E. Enuresis in neglected children. *American Journal of Diseases of Children,* 1940, **59**, 490–496.

White, M. A thousand consecutive cases of enuresis: Results of treatment. *Child and Family,* 1971, **10**, 198–209.

Wickes, J.G. Treatment of persistent enuresis with the electric buzzer. In R. Ulrich, T. Stachnick and J. Malery (eds.), *Control of Human Behavior.* Glenview, Ill. Scott Foresman, 1966.

Wilkins-Jensen, K. Nocturnal bed-wetting: An attempt to treat school children with Banthine and Probanthine. *Acta Paediatricia,* 1959, **118**, 78–84.

Winsbury-White, H.P. A study of 310 cases of enuresis treated by dilation, *British Journal of Urology,* 1941, **97**, 98–100.

Woodhese, D.M., Hall, T.C., and Snodgrass, W.T. An effective control of benign enuresis. *Journal of Urology,* 1967, **97**, 98–100.

Yankelovich, Skelly, and White, In *The General Mills American Family Report.* Minneapolis, Minn. 1977.

Yates, A.J. Enuresis and encopresis In A. Yates (ed.), *Behavior Therapy,* New York, Wiley, 1970.

Yates, A.J. *Theory and practice in behavior therapy.* New York, Wiley, 1975.

Yerkes, R.M. and Dobson, J.D. Enuresis. *Journal of Comparative Neurology and Psychology,* 1908, **18**, 459.

Young, G.C. The family history of enuresis. *Journal of the Royal Institute of Public Health,* 1963, August, 197–201.

Young, G.C. A staggered-wakening procedure in the treatment of enuresis. *Medical Officer,* 1964, **111**, 142–143.

Young, G.C. The aetiology of enuresis in terms of learning theory. *Medical Officer,* 1965a, **113**, 19–22.

Young, G.C. Childhood Enuresis. *Midwife and Health Visitor,* 1965b, **1**, 173–176.

Young, G.C. Personality factors and the treatment of enuresis. *Behaviour Research and Therapy,* 1965c, **3 (2)**, 103–105.

Young, G.C. The problem of enuresis. *British Journal of Hospital Medicine,* 1969, **2**, 628–632.

Young, G.C. and Morgan, R.T.T. Non-attending enuretic children. *Community Medicine,* 1972a, **127**, 155–159.

Young, G.C. and Morgan, R.T.T. Overlearning in the conditioning treatment of enuresis: A long-term follow-up study. *Behaviour Research and Therapy,* 1972 (b), **10**, 409–410.

Young, G.C. and Morgan, R.T.T. Analysis of factors associated with the extinction of a conditioned response. *Behaviour Research and Therapy,* 1973a, **11**, 219–222.

Young, G.C. and Morgan, R.T.T. Rapidity of response to the treatment of enuresis. *Developmental Medicine and Child Neurology,* 1973b, **15**, 448–496.

Young, G.C. and Morgan, R.T.T. Conditioning techniques and enuresis. *Medical Journal of Australia,* 1973c, **2**, 329–332.

Young, G.C. and Turner, R.K. CNS stimulant drugs and conditioning treatment of nocturnal enuresis. *Behaviour Research and Therapy,* 1965, **3**, 93–101.

Zaleski, A., Gerrard, J.W. and Shokeir, M.H. Nocturnal enuresis: The importance of a small bladder capacity. In I. Kolvin, R.C. MacKeith, and S.R. Meadows (eds.), *Bladder control and enuresis,* 1973 Philadelphia, Lippincott.

Zaleski, A., Shokeir, M.K. and Gerrard, J.W. Enuresis: Familial incidence and relationship to allergic disorders. *Canadian Medical Association Journal,* 1972, **106**, 31–38.

Zielinski, R. 500 bed-wetters treated as inpatients. *Praxis der Kinderpsychologie und Kinderpsychiatrie,* 1968, **17** (5), 170–172.

Zufael, R.C. Adult male enuresis: A study of 200 cases. *Journal of Urology,* 1953, **70**, 894–897.

Index